PARAMEDIC EXAM
FLASHCARDS

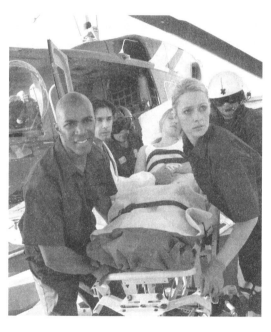

Jeffrey Lindsey, Ph.D., PM, EFO
Coordinator/Lecturer
University of Florida
Gainesville, FL

Research & Education Association
Visit our website at: www.rea.com

Research & Education Association
61 Ethel Road West
Piscataway, New Jersey 08854
E-mail: info@rea.com

Paramedic Exam Flashcard Book
with Online Practice Exam

Printed in the United States of America

ISBN-13: 978-0-7386-1177-8
ISBN-10: 0-7386-1177-8

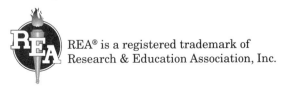

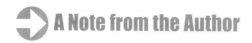 **A Note from the Author**

Serving the public as a paramedic is a rewarding career for anyone who wants to become a first responder. When paramedics respond to a call, they must be prepared for anything and know how to act quickly and safely when someone's life is in their hands.

Paramedics have a great responsibility to the public and must demonstrate their knowledge of certain requirements before receiving certification. In most states, candidates must complete a training program and pass the National Registry of Emergency Medical Technicians (NREMT) Paramedic exam.

Certification as a Nationally Registered Paramedic (NRP) requires that you pass both a cognitive and a psychomotor test. The computer-adaptive multiple-choice cognitive test contains 80 to 150 questions. You will have 2 hours and 30 minutes to complete the exam.

As you prepare for the cognitive test, keep in mind that the key to selecting the correct answer is to read the question carefully and think about what the question is asking. I advise my students to regard the question as a snapshot of the incident. What is happening at the scene? What should you do to help? How would you handle the situation?

The practical, or "hands-on," psychomotor exam, tests your skills in a scenario-type format. To learn more about the specific requirements for this exam, contact your state EMS office or course instructor. For additional information about the Paramedic certification exam, visit *www.nremt.org.*

Taking the Paramedic certification exam can be challenging. You need to prepare yourself by studying your textbook in addition to practicing with REA's *Paramedic Exam Flashcard Book* and online test. Set aside plenty of time, focus on any areas where you feel you need extra review, and relax before the exam.

Being a paramedic is a profession like no other. I wish you the very best on the exam and your career in EMS!

Jeffrey Lindsey, Ph.D., PM, EFO

About This Book

If you are currently enrolled in a paramedic certification program and are getting ready to take the NREMT Paramedic exam, our *Paramedic Exam Flashcard Book* will help you prepare.

Nationally recognized EMT expert Dr. Jeffrey Lindsey gives you 350 practice questions that cover the spectrum of EMS care: airway, respiration and ventilation; cardiology and resuscitation; trauma; medical and obstetrics/gynecology; and EMS operations.

The book presents NREMT-style scenarios designed to prepare you for the types of questions you'll face on the actual exam. Look for the test-category icon on each question to help focus your study on the areas where you need the most review. A complete subject index provides fast access to the full range of Paramedic topics covered.

When you're confident that you have learned the material in the book, go to the REA Study Center (*www.rea.com/studycenter*), take our online Paramedic practice test, and see how well you score. This 100-question test features automatic scoring and diagnostic feedback that identifies any areas in need of further review, helping to ensure that you are ready for test day.

Also at the REA Study Center, you'll find seven invaluable medical reference charts that you can return to time and again:

- Anatomy I
- Anatomy II
- Medical Abbreviations
- Medical Terms: The Basics
- Medical Terms: The Body
- Muscular System
- Skeletal System

These charts provide quick, easy access to important facts you need to know and are great for last-minute review.

Good luck on the exam!

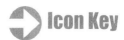

Icon Key

Use these handy icons to locate questions by subject:

	Airway & Breathing Questions about the human pulmonary system, which includes breathing, the mouth, nose, trachea, and the lungs
	**Cardiology** Questions about the heart, particularly its structure, function, and disorders
	Legal Questions about legal concerns
	Medical Questions about medical practices, treatments, and procedures
	Obstetrics & Pediatrics Obstetrics questions on the care of women during pregnancy, childbirth, and the recuperative period following delivery; pediatrics questions on the care of infants and children
	Scene Size-Up Questions on procedures to be employed upon arrival at trauma scene
	Trauma Questions about serious injuries, severe shocks to the body, and appropriate medical treatment

About the Author

Dr. Jeffrey Lindsey has been involved in the emergency services industry since 1980, as a firefighter, fire chief, paramedic, 911 dispatcher, member of national and local safety advisory councils, and he is currently paying it forward as an educator. He is the Coordinator/Lecturer of the Fire Emergency Science program at the University of Florida, and Chief Learning Officer for the Health & Safety Institute.

Dr. Lindsey holds a doctorate and master's degree in Curriculum and Instruction, a bachelor's degree in Fire and Safety Engineering, and an associate's degree in Paramedic. He also achieved the Chief Fire Officer designation and completed the Executive Fire Officer program. He was the 2011 recipient of the James O. Page EMS award, given annually to an individual who has had a positive, national impact on fire-service EMS management and leadership.

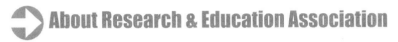
About Research & Education Association

Founded in 1959, Research & Education Association (REA) is dedicated to publishing the finest and most effective educational materials — including study guides and test preps — for students in middle school, high school, college, graduate school, and beyond.

Today, REA's wide-ranging catalog is a leading resource for teachers, students, and professionals. Visit *www.rea.com* to see a complete listing of all our titles.

Acknowledgments

We would like to thank Larry B. Kling, Vice President, Editorial, for his overall direction; Pam Weston, Publisher, for setting the quality standards for production integrity and managing the publication to completion; John Cording, Vice President, Technology, for coordinating the design and development of the REA Study Center; Kelli A. Wilkins, Managing Editor, for project management; Claudia Petrilli, Senior Graphic Designer, for designing our cover; Kathy Caratozzolo of Caragraphics for typesetting the manuscript; Stephanie Reymann for creating the index; and Nimish Mehta, MD, FAAEM and the Young Physicians Section of AAEM for ensuring the technical accuracy of this book.

Questions

Which of the following statements is (are) true?

(A) Criminal law prosecutes people for violating laws intended to protect society.

(B) Civil law deals with conflicts between two parties.

(C) Both A and B are correct

(D) Neither A nor B is correct

Your Answer _____

Which of the following scenarios is an example of malfeasance?

(A) A paramedic assaults a patient.

(B) A paramedic inadvertently intubates a patient's esophagus, fails to confirm tube placement, and leaves the tube in place.

(C) A paramedic fails to fully immobilize a collision patient who is complaining of neck and back pain.

(D) None of the above.

Your Answer _____

Correct Answers

A–1

(C) Criminal law is the part of the legal system that deals with wrongs committed against society or its members; examples are homicide and theft. Civil law is the part of the legal system that deals with conflicts. A civil case usually results in a monetary amount being paid to settle the case rather than disciplinary action, like prison time.

A–2

(A) Malfeasance is the performance of a wrongful or unlawful act or the performance of a legal act in a manner that is harmful or injurious. Nonfeasance is the failure to perform a required act or duty.

Questions

Which of the following best describes a paramedic operating within the scope of practice?

(A) A paramedic is on the scene of a motor vehicle accident. The patient is 8 months pregnant, in critical condition, and probably going to die. A fetal heartbeat is evident. The paramedic elects to do a cesarean section on the scene to save the baby. This procedure is not part of the EMS agency's protocols.

(B) A paramedic is on the scene of a patient having chest pain. The patient has been having chest pain for the past hour. The paramedic elects to give the patient a spray of the patient's nitroglycerin.

(C) A paramedic is en route to the hospital with an elderly patient. The patient goes into cardiac arrest. The patient's family stated not to do CPR on the patient should he go into cardiac arrest.

(D) A paramedic is on the scene of a cardiac patient having chest pain. The patient weighs approximately 100 kilograms. The online medical control doctor orders 1 gram of lidocaine.

Your Answer _____

_____

Fast Fact

In the United States there are 17,000 transporting ambulance services (includes fire departments).

Correct Answers

(B)   It is acceptable, and within a paramedic's scope of practice, to administer the patient's nitroglycerin. It is not acceptable to do a cesarean section, unless it is part of the EMS agency's protocols. While such occurrences have been reported, it is by no means an acceptable procedure. It is perfectly acceptable to withhold CPR if the paramedic has the appropriate DNR paperwork. It is not within the scope of practice to make the decision based on a family member's request. Finally, if a paramedic gets an order (that is clearly incorrect), the paramedic needs to clarify the order with the online medical control doctor.

Career Pulse

NREMT computer-based exams are constructed to ensure that each candidate receives a distribution of items from six major categories: Airway & Breathing, Cardiology, Medical, Trauma, OB/Gyn/Peds, and Operations.

Questions

When delivering your report to the receiving hospital over the radio, you should report all of the following EXCEPT

(A) your unit number.
(B) the patient's sex and age.
(C) the patient's name.
(D) the patient's current illness.

Your Answer _____

_____

In which of the following scenarios would express consent be applicable?

(A) A 27-year-old female is unresponsive and having seizures.
(B) A 33-year-old male is having a psychiatric emergency.
(C) A 14-year-old male fell off a bike and sustained a laceration to the left knee.
(D) A 52-year-old female is awake and alert but having chest pain.

Your Answer _____

_____

Correct Answers

A–4

(C) When giving a report to the receiving hospital by radio you should give the following information: your unit number, your level of certification, ETA, age and sex of the patient, chief complaint, brief pertinent history of the present illness, major past illnesses, mental status, baseline vital signs, pertinent findings, medical care given, and response to the medical treatment. You should never give the patient's name over the radio. This may be seen as a breach of patient confidentiality.

A–5

(D) Express consent is when a patient gives verbal, nonverbal, or written consent to receive medical care. The 52-year-old female having chest pain can give express consent because she is awake and alert. A patient who is unresponsive cannot give express consent. A patient having a psychiatric emergency is not mentally able to give express consent. The 14-year-old male is a minor and therefore cannot give express consent unless he has a life-threatening emergency.

Questions

Which of the following is a legal document that allows people to specify the kinds of medical treatments they wish to receive when the need arises?

(A) Living will
(B) Advance directive
(C) DNR
(D) Health care surrogate

Your Answer _____

Q–7

Which of the following is a legal document, usually signed by the patient and a physician, that indicates to medical personnel which, if any, life-saving measures to take when the patient's heart and respiratory functions have ceased?

(A) Living will
(B) Advance directive
(C) DNR
(D) Health care surrogate

Your Answer _____

Correct Answers

(A)   A living will is a legal document that allows people to specify the kinds of medical treatments they wish to receive when the need arises. An advance directive is a document created to ensure that certain treatment choices are honored when a patient is unconscious or otherwise unable to express a treatment choice. A DNR is a legal document, usually signed by the patient and a physician, that indicates to medical personnel which, if any, life-saving measures to take when the patient's heart and respiratory functions have ceased. A health care surrogate is appointed to make medical decisions for the patient.

(C)   A DNR is a legal document, usually signed by the patient and a physician, that indicates to medical personnel which, if any, life-saving measures should be taken when the patient's heart and respiratory functions have ceased. A living will is a legal document that allows people to specify the kinds of medical treatments they wish to receive when the need arises. An advance directive is a document created to ensure that certain treatment choices are honored when a patient is unconscious or otherwise unable to express a treatment choice. A health care surrogate is appointed to make medical decisions for the patient.

Questions

There are four fundamental principles, or values, applied to resolving problems in bioethics today. They are all the following EXCEPT

(A) beneficence
(B) malfeasance
(C) autonomy
(D) judgment

Your Answer _____

The genetic material deoxyribonucleic acid and the enzymes necessary for its replication are found in the

(A) endoplasmic reticulum
(B) Golgi apparatus
(C) organelles
(D) nucleus

Your Answer _____

Correct Answers

A–8

(D) Beneficence means to do good, malfeasance means doing harm, and autonomy refers to a competent adult patient's right to determine what happens to his or her body. These are three of the four fundamental principles or values. The fourth principle is justice: the paramedic's obligation to treat all patients fairly. Judgment is not one of the four.

A–9

(D) The nucleus contains deoxyribonucleic acid, or DNA. The endoplasmic reticulum is a network of small channels that have both rough and smooth portions. The Golgi apparatus is located near the nucleus of most cells. Organelles are structures that perform specific functions within a cell.

Questions

Which of the following attacks foreign substances as part of the body's immune response?

(A) Erythrocyte
(B) Lymphocyte
(C) Thrombocyte
(D) Granulocyte

Your Answer _____

Which of the following is a cell that has the ability to ingest other cells and substances such as bacteria and cellular debris?

(A) Phagocyte
(B) Lymphocyte
(C) Cytotoxin
(D) Granulocyte

Your Answer _____

Correct Answers

A–10

(B) A lymphocyte, or white blood cell, attacks foreign substances as part of the body's immune response. Erythrocytes are red blood cells. Thrombocytes are responsible for the initial steps in the clotting cascade. Granulocytes are specific types of white cells with multiple nuclei that aid in fighting off infection.

A–11

(A) A phagocyte is a cell that has the ability to ingest other cells and substances like bacteria and cellular debris. A lymphocyte, or white blood cell, attacks foreign substances as part of the body's immune response. Cytotoxin is a substance that is poisonous to cells. Granulocytes are specific types of white cells with multiple nuclei that aid in fighting infection.

Questions

Which of the following is the most abundant body tissue?

(A) Muscle
(B) Connective
(C) Epithelial
(D) Skeletal

Your Answer _____

The three types of muscle tissue are all the following EXCEPT

(A) cardiac
(B) smooth
(C) autonomic
(D) striated

Your Answer _____

Correct Answers

A–12

(B)   The most abundant tissue in the body is connective tissue.

A–13

(C)   The three types of muscle tissue are cardiac, smooth, and striated.

Questions

Q–14

Which type of muscle encircles the blood vessels?

(A) Cardiac
(B) Smooth
(C) Autonomic
(D) Striated

Your Answer _____

Q–15

The natural tendency of the body to maintain a steady and normal internal environment is called

(A) metabolism
(B) pathophysiological
(C) automenomic
(D) homeostasis

Your Answer _____

Correct Answers

A–14

(B) Smooth muscle is found within the intestines and encircling blood vessels. Cardiac muscle is found only within the heart. Striated or skeletal muscle allows for movement, and unlike cardiac and smooth muscle, is mostly under voluntary control.

A–15

(D) Homeostasis is the natural tendency of the body to maintain a steady and normal internal environment. Metabolism is the total change that takes place to generate energy for physiological processes. There is no such thing as automenomic.

Questions

Match each of the following terms to the correct definition.

Q–16   Atrophy

Q–17   Hypertrophy

Q–18   Dilation

Q–19   Hyperplasia

Q–20   Mitosis

Q–21   Metaplasia

Q–22   Dysplasia

(A) An abnormal enlargement resulting from pathology

(B) A change in cell size, shape, or appearance caused by an external stressor

(C) A decrease in cell size resulting from a decreased workload

(D) An increase in cell size resulting from an increased workload

(E) The process by which cells divide

(F) The replacement of one type of cell by another type of cell that is not normal for that tissue

(G) An increase in the number of cells resulting from an increased workload

Your Answer _____

_____

Fast Fact

In the United States there are 26,000 fire departments (most of which provide some sort of EMS and about half of which offer ambulance transport).

Correct Answers

A–16
(C) Atrophy is a decrease in cell size resulting from a decreased workload.

A–17
(D) Hypertrophy is an increase in cell size resulting from an increased workload.

A–18
(A) Dilation is an abnormal enlargement resulting from pathology, as sometimes occurs in the heart. Dilation can also be a normal process, such as papillary dilation when you enter a dark room.

A–19
(G) Hyperplasia is an increase in number of cells resulting from an increased workload or from a precancerous condition.

A–20
(E) Mitosis is the process by which cells divide.

A–21
(F) Metaplasia is the replacement of one type of cell by another type of cell that is not normal for that tissue.

A–22
(B) Dysplasia is a change in cell size, shape, or appearance caused by an external stressor.

Questions

Q–23

A patient is in an anaerobic metabolic state. This state is characterized by

(A) a marked decrease in cellular ATP production and a decrease in the production of lactic acid
(B) a marked decrease in cellular ATP production and an increase in the production of lactic acid
(C) a marked increase in cellular ATP production and a decrease in the production of lactic acid
(D) a marked increase in cellular ATP production and an increase in the production of lactic acid

Your Answer _____

Q–24

A cell membrane has fewer particles on one side compared with the other side. The side with fewer particles is

(A) the osmotic gradient
(B) hypertonic
(C) hypotonic
(D) isotonic

Your Answer _____

Correct Answers

(B) A patient in an anaerobic state (lacking oxygen) has a marked decrease in cellular ATP production and an increase in the production of harmful acids, primarily lactic acid.

(C) A cell membrane with fewer particles on one side than on the other side is hypotonic. If a cell membrane has more particles on one side than on the other, it is hypertonic. An isotonic cell membrane has equal concentrations of solute molecules or particles on both sides. The osmotic gradient is the difference in concentration between solutions on opposite sides of a semipermeable membrane. Particles or solutes generally travel from an area of higher concentration (hypertonic) to an area of lower concentration (hypotonic).

Questions

Match each of the following terms to the correct definition.

Q–25 Plasma

Q–26 Erythrocytes

Q–27 Leukocytes

Q–28 Thrombocytes

Q–29 Hemoglobin

Q–30 Hematocrit

(A) Platelets, which are important in blood clotting

(B) The liquid part of the blood

(C) The percentage of the blood occupied by red blood cells

(D) Transport oxygen to cells

(E) An iron-based compound that binds with oxygen and transports it to the cells

(F) Play a key role in the immune system and inflammatory response

Your Answer _____

_____

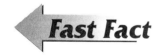

In the United States there are over 52,000 ambulances.

Correct Answers

A–25

(B) Plasma is the liquid part of the blood.

A–26

(D) Erythrocytes, or red blood cells, contain hemoglobin and transport oxygen to the cells.

A–27

(F) Leukocytes, or white blood cells, play a key role in the immune system and inflammatory response.

A–28

(A) Thrombocytes are platelets, which are important in blood clotting.

A–29

(E) Hemoglobin is an iron-based compound that binds with oxygen and transports it to the cells.

A–30

(C) Hematocrit is the percentage of the blood occupied by red blood cells, or erythrocytes.

Career Pulse

The number of items from each category of the NREMT computer-based exams is determined by an examination test plan (also known as a blueprint), which has been approved by the NREMT Board of Directors.

Questions

A patient is hyperventilating. In this situation, the patient is most likely in

(A) respiratory acidosis
(B) respiratory alkalosis
(C) metabolic acidosis
(D) metabolic alkalosis

Your Answer _____

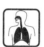

Which of the following conditions would, on rare occasions, require treatment with an IV bolus of sodium bicarbonate?

(A) Respiratory acidosis
(B) Respiratory alkalosis
(C) Metabolic acidosis
(D) Metabolic alkalosis

Your Answer _____

Correct Answers

A–31

(B) This patient is most likely in respiratory alkalosis, which results from an excessive elimination of carbon dioxide caused by an increased respiratory rate. Respiratory acidosis is abnormal retention of carbon dioxide resulting from hypoventilation. Metabolic acidosis is an increase in the production of acids during metabolism that can be caused by vomiting, diarrhea, diabetes, medication, or other conditions. Metabolic alkalosis is caused by an increase in plasma bicarbonate resulting from diuresis, vomiting, ingestion of too much sodium bicarbonate, or other causes.

A–32

(C) A patient in metabolic acidosis, on rare occasions, would be given an IV bolus of sodium bicarbonate.

Questions

You arrive on the scene to find a 54-year-old male complaining of severe shortness of breath. You auscultate his breath sounds and hear crackles bilaterally. He states that he has pink, frothy sputum. The patient is most likely in

(A) cardiogenic shock
(B) septic shock
(C) hypovolemic shock
(D) neurogenic shock

Your Answer _____

_____

Your patient is warm with red skin. The patient's pulse is 60, respirations are 20, and blood pressure is 80/40. This patient is most likely suffering from

(A) cardiogenic shock
(B) septic shock
(C) anaphylactic shock
(D) neurogenic shock

Your Answer _____

_____

Correct Answers

A–33

(A) This patient is likely in cardiogenic shock. Cardiogenic shock is characterized by pulmonary edema. The pink, frothy sputum and crackles on auscultation are characteristic of pulmonary edema.

A–34

(D) Patients in neurogenic shock typically have reflex bradycardia and hypotension as a result of vasodilation. Although the blood vessels dilate, the blood volume stays constant, resulting in hypotension. The patient's skin is also warm and dry because of vasodilation and disruption of nerves to the skin.

Questions

Which of the following is NOT a complication of peripheral IV access?

(A) Pyrogenic reaction
(B) Thrombophlebitis
(C) Necrosis
(D) Catheter at a gate

Your Answer _____

Which of the following statements about the location for intraosseous site accesses is correct?

(A) Pediatric, adult, and geriatric accesses use the proximal tibia.
(B) Pediatric and geriatric accesses use the proximal tibia. Adult access uses the distal tibia.
(C) Pediatric access uses the proximal tibia. Adult and geriatric accesses use the distal tibia.
(D) Pediatric, adult, and geriatric accesses use the distal tibia.

Your Answer _____

Correct Answers

A–35

(D) A pyrogenic reaction occurs in the presence of foreign proteins capable of producing a febrile response. Thrombophlebitis is inflammation of a vein and occurs particularly in patients undergoing long-term IV therapy. Necrosis is the sloughing off of dead tissue. The catheter at a gate is common but not a complication. The catheter needs to be pulled back from the gate, allowing the flow to resume without incident.

A–36

(C) Pediatric access uses the proximal tibia. Adult and geriatric accesses use the distal tibia.

Questions

911

Which of the following is NOT a contraindication to intraosseous placement?

(A) Fracture to the tibia or femur on the side of access
(B) Osteogenesis imperfecta
(C) Osteoporosis
(D) No peripheral IV line

Your Answer _____

Convert 5.8 milligrams to micrograms.

(A) 5,800
(B) 0.0000058
(C) 0.0058
(D) 5,800,000

Your Answer _____

Correct Answers

A–37

$\boxed{911}$

(D) Fracture of the tibia or femur on the side of access, osteogenesis imperfecta, osteoporosis, and establishment of a peripheral IV line are contraindications to intraosseous placement.

A–38

(A) First, convert 5.8 milligrams to grams: 5.8 mg / 1000 = 0.0058 g. Then convert 0.0058 grams to micrograms: 0.0058 g × 1,000,000 = 5,800 mcg.

Questions

Your patient weighs 188 pounds. How much does your patient weigh in kilograms?

(A) 85
(B) 94
(C) 80.5
(D) 85.5

Your Answer _____

You are treating a patient and are ordered to give 2.5 mg of medication subcutaneously. The ampule contains 10 mg of the drug in 2 mL of solution. How much medication should you administer?

(A) 1 mL
(B) 0.25 mL
(C) 2.5 mL
(D) 0.5 mL

Your Answer _____

Correct Answers

A–39

(D) 188 lb / 2.2 = 85.5 kg.

A–40

(D) Volume × Desired dose / Dosage on hand = 2 mL × 2.5 mg / 10 mg = 0.5 mL.

Questions

You are treating a patient weighing 100 kg with hypoperfusion. You are ordered to give 5 mcg of dopamine. Your IV concentration is 400 mg dopamine in a 500 mL bag of IV solution. You have a microdrip administration set. How many drops per minute should you administer?

(A) 15
(B) 37.5
(C) 22.5
(D) 30

Your Answer _____

Decreased CO_2 elimination (that is, increased CO_2 levels in the blood) results from decreased alveolar ventilation. Common causes include hypoventilation caused by any of the following EXCEPT

(A) increased respirations resulting from drugs
(B) airway obstruction
(C) impairment of the respiratory muscles
(D) obstructive disease such as asthma or emphysema

Your Answer _____

Correct Answers

A–41

(B) (Volume on hand × Drip factor × Desired dose) / Dosage on hand = Drops per minute = (500 mL × 60 gtts/mL × 5 mcg) / 400 mg = 37.5 gtts/min.

A–42

(A) Decreased CO_2 elimination (that is, increased CO_2 level in the blood) results from decreased alveolar ventilation. The common cause is hypoventilation caused by respiratory depression resulting from drugs, airway obstruction, impairment of the respiratory muscles, or an obstructive disease such as asthma or emphysema.

Questions

Deep, slow or rapid, and gasping breathing, commonly found in diabetic ketoacidosis, is a sign and symptom of

(A) Cheyne-Stokes respiration
(B) Biot respiration
(C) Kussmaul respiration
(D) agonal respiration

Your Answer _____

Your patient has Cheyne-Stokes respiration. What condition might this type of breathing indicate?

(A) Diabetic acidosis
(B) Brain stem injury
(C) Increased intracranial pressure
(D) Brain anoxia

Your Answer _____

Correct Answers

A–43

(C) Kussmaul respiration is deep, slow or rapid, and gasping breathing commonly found in patients with diabetic ketoacidosis. Cheyne-Stokes respiration is breathing that gets progressively deeper and faster, alternating gradually with shallow, slower breathing. Biot respiration is breathing with an irregular pattern of rate and depth and sudden, periodic episodes of apnea. Agonal respiration is shallow, slow or infrequent breathing.

A–44

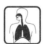

(B) Cheyne-Stokes respiration indicates brain stem injury. Kussmaul respiration indicates diabetic acidosis. Biot respiration and central neurogenic hyperventilation indicate increased intracranial pressure. Brain anoxia is indicated by agonal respiration.

Questions

Your patient has a harsh, high-pitched sound on inhalation. The patient also has laryngeal edema. What would you expect to hear when listening to breath sounds?

(A) Snoring
(B) Stridor
(C) Wheezing
(D) Rhonchi

Your Answer _____

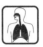

Your patient has a fine, bubbling sound on inspiration. You would classify this breath sound as

(A) crackles
(B) stridor
(C) wheezing
(D) rhonchi

Your Answer _____

Correct Answers

A–45

(B) You would hear stridor with this patient. Snoring is a result of partial obstruction of the upper airway. Wheezing is a musical, squeaking, or whistling sound heard on inspiration and/or expiration, associated with bronchiolar constriction. Rhonchi are coarse, rattling noises heard on inspiration and associated with inflammation, mucus, or fluid in the bronchioles.

A–46

(A) Crackles is a fine, bubbling sound on inspiration. Stridor is a harsh, high-pitched sound heard on inspiration. Wheezing is a musical, squeaking, or whistling sound heard on inspiration and/or expiration, associated with bronchiolar constriction. Rhonchi are coarse, rattling noises heard on inspiration and associated with inflammation, mucus, or fluid in the bronchioles.

Questions

Which of the following is a normal SaO$_2$ range?

(A) 88%–100%
(B) 90%–100%
(C) 95%–99%
(D) 90%–99%

Your Answer _____

_____

You need to help prevent regurgitation and reduce gastric distention on a patient you are ventilating. To do this, you would

(A) do a finger sweep
(B) apply pressure to the abdomen
(C) ventilate the patient faster
(D) do the Sellick maneuver

Your Answer _____

_____

Correct Answers

A–47

(C) The normal SaO_2 range is 95%–99%.

A–48

(D) To prevent regurgitation and reduce gastric distention, you should perform the Sellick maneuver. This maneuver is performed by applying gentle pressure over the cricoid cartilage, causing the esophagus to become occluded.

Questions

Which of the following is NOT an advantage of using a nasopharyngeal airway?

(A) It does not isolate the trachea.
(B) It can be rapidly inserted and safely placed blindly.
(C) You may use it in the presence of a gag reflex in a patient who is awake.
(D) You may suction through it.

Your Answer _____

All the following are disadvantages of an oropharyngeal airway EXCEPT

(A) it does not isolate the trachea
(B) it is easily dislodged
(C) return of the gag reflex may produce vomiting
(D) air can pass around and through the device

Your Answer _____

Correct Answers

A–49

(A) Not isolating the trachea is a disadvantage of the nasopharyngeal airway.

A–50

(D) The ability of air to pass around and through the device is an advantage of using the oropharyngeal airway.

Questions

Q–51

Which of the following is NOT an advantage of endotracheal intubation?

(A) It isolates the trachea and permits complete control of the airway.
(B) It requires direct visualization of the vocal cords.
(C) It impedes gastric distention by channeling air directly into the trachea.
(D) It offers a direct route for suctioning of the respiratory passages.

Your Answer _____

_____

Q–52

You have just intubated your patient. Which scenario would indicate a successful tracheal intubation?

(A) Gurgling sounds over the epigastrium with each breath delivered
(B) A falling pulse oximetry reading
(C) A persistent air leak, despite inflation of the tube's distal cuff
(D) Color change with a colorimetric ETCO2 detector

Your Answer _____

_____

Correct Answers

(B) A disadvantage of endotracheal intubation is that it requires direct visualization of the vocal cords via laryngoscopy. The advantages of endotracheal intubation are that it isolates the trachea and permits complete control of the airway, it impedes gastric distention by channeling air directly into the trachea, it eliminates the need to maintain a mask seal, and it offers a direct route for suctioning of the respiratory passages.

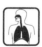

(D) Color change with a colorimetric $ETCO_2$ detector is one indication of a tracheal intubation. The other selections are indicators of esophageal intubation. In addition, positive lung sounds, absent sounds over the abdomen, chest rise and fall, and fogging of the tube are other indicators of tracheal intubation.

Questions

Many complications are associated with endotracheal intubation. One complication is dental injury and soft tissue lacerations. Which scenario would eliminate this complication?

(A) When inserting the blade into the mouth and pharynx, guide it gently into place, avoiding pressure on the teeth.

(B) When manipulating the jaw anteriorly, use gentle traction downward and toward the head, rather than rotating and flexing your wrist.

(C) Both A and B.

(D) Neither A nor B.

Your Answer _____

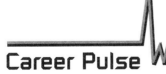

Career Pulse

The NREMT examination test plan is developed based upon the result of the EMT-Paramedic Practice Analysis that is conducted every five years.

Correct Answers

A–53

(A) When inserting the blade into the mouth and pharynx, guide it gently into place, avoiding pressure on the teeth. When manipulating the jaw anteriorly, use gentle traction upward and toward the feet, rather than rotating and flexing your wrist; this technique helps eliminate dental injury and soft tissue lacerations.

Fast Fact

In the United States there are more than 600,000 EMTs and 142,000 paramedics.

Questions

You have just intubated your patient. You auscultate the patient's breath sounds. You hear good breath sounds over the right side but not the left. Which scenario is most likely the cause of this finding?

(A) Tension pneumothorax
(B) Right mainstem bronchus intubation
(C) Left mainstem bronchus intubation
(D) Esophageal intubation

Your Answer _____

Your EMT partner is ventilating the patient you intubated. Your partner tells you that it is becoming more difficult to ventilate the patient. You notice the trachea is deviated to the left and breath sounds are absent over the right side. You would suspect

(A) tension pneumothorax
(B) right mainstem bronchus intubation
(C) left mainstem bronchus intubation
(D) esophageal intubation

Your Answer _____

Correct Answers

A–54

(B) The most common cause of breath sounds on the right side and not on the left side is right mainstem bronchus intubation. To correct this problem, you need to deflate the cuff and withdraw the tube a centimeter or so until you hear breath sounds on both sides of the chest. Other, more rare causes of absent breath sounds on the left side are a tension pneumothorax on the left side, a left side pneumonectomy, and an obstructed left mainstem bronchus.

A–55

(A) This patient is exhibiting all the signs and symptoms of a tension pneumothorax. You would need to do a right-sided chest decompression.

Questions

You are treating a head injury patient who has an altered mental status. The patient's airway needs protection. Which scenario would be the best method to protect this patient's airway?

(A) Insert a nasopharyngeal airway
(B) Administer 15 LPM of oxygen through a nonre-breather mask
(C) Perform a rapid-sequence intubation
(D) Ventilate the patient with a bag valve mask

Your Answer _____

Which scenario is NOT an indication for a rapid-sequence intubation?

(A) 62-year-old male with impending respiratory failure as a result of congestive heart failure (CHF)
(B) 28-year-old female with acute airway disorder as a result of facial burns
(C) 19-year-old anaphylaxis patient with urticaria
(D) 36-year-old patient with drug overdose and altered mental status who has vomited

Your Answer _____

Correct Answers

A–56

(C) The best method to protect this patient is to do a rapid-sequence intubation. The other methods are possible but do not afford the protection that intubation provides.

A–57

(C) A rapid-sequence intubation is indicated with any patient who has impending respiratory failure owing to intrinsic pulmonary disease such as chronic obstructive pulmonary disease (COPD), CHF, asthma, or pneumonia. Other indications include an acute airway disorder that threatens airway patency, such as facial burns; laryngeal or upper airway trauma; and altered mental status with significant risk of vomiting and aspiration, as in head trauma, drug or alcohol intoxication, or status epilepticus.

Questions

Which statement is true regarding pediatric intubation?

(A) The tongue is proportional to the oropharynx.

(B) The epiglottis is floppy and round.

(C) The glottic opening is lower and more posterior in the neck.

(D) The widest part of the airway is at the cricoid cartilage.

Your Answer _____

_____

911

Your patient has a possible spinal injury. You cannot get the patient's mouth to open. No facial injuries are apparent. The best airway for this patient is

(A) orotracheal intubation

(B) oropharyngeal airway

(C) nasotracheal intubation

(D) nasopharyngeal airway

Your Answer _____

_____

Correct Answers

A–58

(B) The epiglottis is floppy and round. The tongue is larger in relation to the oropharynx. The glottic opening is higher and more anterior in the neck. The narrowest part of the airway is at the cricoid cartilage.

A–59

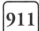

(C) The best choice for this patient is a nasotracheal intubation. A nasotracheal intubation can be performed in a patient with spinal injuries and no severe facial injuries or fractures. In addition, it is much easier to do a nasotracheal intubation on a patient who still has a gag reflex. Because this patient's mouth was clenched shut, an orotracheal intubation would be difficult.

Questions

All the following are complications of a needle cricothyrotomy EXCEPT

(A) barotrauma from underinflation

(B) excessive bleeding as a result of improper catheter placement

(C) airway obstruction from compression of the trachea secondary to excessive bleeding or subcutaneous air

(D) hypoventilation from the use of improper equipment, incorrect use of the jet ventilator, or misplacement of the catheter

Your Answer _____

_____

A stoma is

(A) an airway used for patients with a blocked airway

(B) an opening in the anterior neck that connects the trachea with ambient air

(C) a trachea tube used to secure the airway of a patient who has facial trauma

(D) none of the above

Your Answer _____

_____

Correct Answers

A–60

(A) All are true except that barotrauma is caused by overinflation, not underinflation.

A–61

(B) A stoma is an opening in the anterior neck that connects the trachea with ambient air.

Questions

You are suctioning a patient who has vomited. You should suction no longer than

(A) 5 seconds
(B) 10 seconds
(C) 15 seconds
(D) 20 seconds

Your Answer _____

Which of the following is NOT part of assessing the history of a present illness?

(A) Radiation
(B) Pertinent negatives
(C) Provocation
(D) Medications

Your Answer _____

Correct Answers

A–62

(B) Suctioning deprives a patient of oxygen. Therefore, you should suction no longer than 10 seconds.

A–63

(D) Medications are included in an assessment of a patient's medical history. The elements of a history of a present illness can be remembered by the mnemonic OPQRST: onset, provocation, quality, radiation, severity, and time. Associated symptoms and pertinent negatives are also elements of the history of a present illness.

Questions

Which of the following is a pertinent negative?

(A) You are treating a patient who is complaining of chest pain but denying any shortness of breath.

(B) You are treating a patient who has a head injury and has lost consciousness.

(C) You are treating a patient who is short of breath and has a productive cough.

(D) You are treating a patient who is having abdominal pain but denies having a headache.

Your Answer _____

It is important to assess a patient's medical history. Which of the following is NOT part of a medical history?

(A) Surgeries and hospitalizations

(B) Medications

(C) Medical insurance

(D) Medical problems

Your Answer _____

Correct Answers

(A) When a patient is having chest pain but does not have shortness of breath, the absence of shortness of breath is important to note and a pertinent negative. Choices B and C describe positive occurrences. Typically, headache and abdominal pain are unrelated conditions; therefore, D is not a pertinent negative.

(C) Medical history is the general state of the patient's health, pertinent childhood and adult diseases or medical problems, surgeries and hospitalizations, medications, and known allergies. The patient's medical insurance is not pertinent to the medical history.

Questions

Q–66

Your patient is complaining of ringing in the ears. This condition is called

(A) tympany
(B) hyper-resonance
(C) rhinitis
(D) tinnitus

Your Answer _____

Q–67

Which of the following refers to the number of viable births a woman has had?

(A) Gravida
(B) Para
(C) Abortion
(D) Pregnancy

Your Answer _____

Correct Answers

A–66

(D)   Tympany and hyper-resonance are percussion sounds. Rhinitis is a runny nose. Tinnitus is ringing of the ears.

A–67

(B)   Para is the number of viable births. Gravida is how many times a woman has been pregnant. Abortion is the loss of the fetus.

Questions

You are examining your patient, who reports coughing up blood. The term for coughing up blood is

(A) hematuria
(B) hemoptysis
(C) hematemesis
(D) hematoma

Your Answer _____

Your elderly patient has had a gradual deterioration of her mental status over several months. Her friend says that she was diagnosed with a structural neurological disease. This patient most likely has

(A) depression
(B) delirium
(C) dementia
(D) distress

Your Answer _____

Correct Answers

(B) Hemoptysis is coughing up blood. Hematuria is blood in the urine. Hematemesis is vomiting blood. Hematoma is a collection of blood under the surface of the skin.

(C) Dementia is a gradual deterioration of mental status usually associated with structural neurological disease. Depression is a mood disorder characterized by hopelessness and malaise. Delirium is an acute alteration in mental functioning that is often reversible.

Questions

Which of the following is NOT a technique of the physical examination?

(A) Inspection
(B) Palpation
(C) Percussion
(D) Regulation

Your Answer _____

You are assessing a patient's pulse. The pulse is bounding. This would be the

(A) quality
(B) rhythm
(C) rate
(D) pressure

Your Answer _____

Correct Answers

A–70

(D) Inspection, palpation, percussion, and auscultation are the techniques of the physical examination.

A–71

(A) Bounding is the quality of the pulse. The rhythm is the pattern and equality of intervals between the beats. The rate is how fast the heart is beating. The pressure is the amount of pressure against the vessel walls.

Questions

Match each of the following terms to the correct pulse location.

Q–72   Temporal

Q–73   Carotid

Q–74   Brachial

Q–75   Radial

Q–76   Ulnar

Q–77   Femoral

Q–78   Popliteal

Q–79   Dorsalis pedis

Q–80   Posterior tibial

(A) Top of foot

(B) Thumb side of wrist

(C) Just below inguinal ligament

(D) Lateral to eye orbit

(E) Just medial to biceps tendon

(F) Behind medial malleolus

(G) Just behind knee

(H) Little-finger side of wrist

(I) Medial to and below angle of jaw

Your Answer _____

Fast Fact

In the United States there are more than 1,009,000 firefighters, many of whom are cross-trained in EMS.

Correct Answers

A–72
(D)   Temporal—lateral to eye orbit

A–73
(I)   Carotid—medial to and below angle of jaw

A–74
(E)   Brachial—just medial to biceps tendon

A–75
(B)   Radial—thumb side of wrist

A–76
(H)   Ulnar—little-finger side of wrist

A–77
(C)   Femoral—just below inguinal ligament

A–78
(G)   Popliteal—just behind knee

A–79
(A)   Dorsalis pedis—top of foot

A–80
(F)   Posterior tibial—behind medial malleolus

Career Pulse

The NREMT randomly surveys hundreds of practicing NREMT-Paramedics. These individuals are asked to provide information about the important tasks that a paramedic performs.

Questions

The normal tidal volume for an average-sized adult at rest is

(A) 250 mL
(B) 500 mL
(C) 750 mL
(D) 1000 mL

Your Answer _____

You are assessing a 26-year-old male patient. The patient is breathing at 8 breaths per minute. The patient's respiratory rate is

(A) tachypnea
(B) eupnea
(C) bradypnea
(D) apnea

Your Answer _____

Correct Answers

A–81

(B)   The tidal volume for an average-sized adult at rest is 500 mL.

A–82

(C)   The normal respiratory rate for an adult is 12 to 20 breaths per minute. Eupnea is a normal breathing rate and pattern. Anything less than 12 is bradypnea. Anything greater than 20 is tachypnea. Apnea is the absence of breathing.

Questions

You are dispatched to a patient who was submerged under-water for 10 minutes. The water temperature is 50°F. You would suspect this patient to be suffering from

(A) hypothermia
(B) hyperthermia
(C) normothermia
(D) hypertension

Your Answer _____

911

Your patient has suffered a brain stem injury. The patient's intracranial pressure is increasing. Which breathing pattern would you expect to see with this injury?

(A) Tachypnea
(B) Bradypnea
(C) Cheyne-Stokes
(D) Apneusis

Your Answer _____

Correct Answers

A–83

(A) This patient would most likely be suffering from hypothermia, or low body temperature. Hyperthermia is elevated body temperature. Normothermia is normal body temperature. Hypertension is high blood pressure.

A–84

(C) With Cheyne-Stokes respiration, the patient's breathing gradually increases and then decreases, with intermittent periods of apnea. This pattern is common in patients with increased intracranial pressure resulting from brain stem injury and can also be seen at high altitudes. Tachypnea is a fast breathing rate. Bradypnea is a slow breathing rate. A patient with apneusis has a prolonged inspiratory phase with shortened expiratory phase; this pattern is common with lesions in the brain stem.

Questions

You are treating a patient with acute renal failure. You would suspect this patient's breathing pattern to be

(A) eupnea
(B) Kussmaul
(C) Cheyne-Stokes
(D) Biot

Your Answer _____

_____

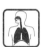

You are treating a patient complaining of trouble breathing. You apply the pulse oximeter. The reading is 89%. Your best course of action would be

(A) remove the device and reapply
(B) begin CPR
(C) begin positive-pressure ventilation
(D) administer 6 LPM of oxygen via nasal cannula

Your Answer _____

_____

Correct Answers

A–85

(B)   A patient in renal failure will most likely exhibit Kussmaul respiration. Patients in metabolic acidosis and diabetic ketoacidosis will also exhibit Kussmaul respiration in an attempt to eliminate excess acids by exhaling carbon dioxide. Eupnea is the normal breathing pattern. With Cheyne-Stokes respiration, the patient experiences a gradual increase and then decrease in breathing, with periods of apnea. Biot respiration is rapid, deep breathing with short pauses between sets and is seen in patients with spinal meningitis and various disorders of the central nervous system.

A–86

(C)   When a patient's pulse oximeter reading drops to 90 or below, the best action is to begin positive-pressure ventilation immediately. Immediate oxygen administration is the next best action.

Questions

Match each of the following lung sounds to the appropriate definition.

Q–87 Rales
Q–88 Wheezes
Q–89 Rhonchi
Q–90 Stridor

(A) Continuous sounds with a lower pitch and a snoring quality
(B) Light, crackling, popping, nonmusical sounds usually heard during inspiration
(C) Predominately inspiratory wheeze associated with laryngeal obstruction
(D) Continuous, high-pitched musical sounds similar to a whistle

Your Answer _____

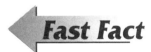

Salaries of paid EMTs and paramedics are generally below $30,000.

Correct Answers

A–87

(B) Rales or crackles are light, crackling, popping, non-musical sounds usually heard during inspiration.

A–88

(D) Wheezes are continuous, high-pitched musical sounds similar to a whistle.

A–89

(A) Rhonchi are continuous sounds with a lower pitch and a snoring quality.

A–90

(C) Stridor is a predominately inspiratory wheeze associated with laryngeal obstruction.

Career Pulse

A committee composed of national experts reviews the results of the data from the NREMT survey and develops a test plan that is approved by the Board of Directors.

Questions

Match each of the cranial nerves to the correct innervation.

Q–91   I, olfactory
Q–92   II, optic
Q–93   III, oculomotor
Q–94   IV, trochlear
Q–95   V, trigeminal
Q–96   VI, abducens
Q–97   VII, facial
Q–98   VIII, acoustic
Q–99   IX, glossopharyngeal
Q–100 X, vagus
Q–101 XI, accessory
Q–102 XII, hypoglossal

(A) Tongue and facial muscles
(B) Superior oblique muscles
(C) Lateral rectus muscle
(D) Tongue
(E) Posterior pharynx
(F) Sight
(G) Chewing muscles
(H) Trapezius muscles
(I) Hearing balance
(J) Taste to posterior tongue, diaphragm
(K) Smell
(L) Pupil constriction

Your Answer _____

_____

Correct Answers

A–91
(K) I, olfactory—smell

A–92
(F) II, optic—sight

A–93
(L) III, oculomotor—pupil constriction

A–94
(B) IV, trochlear—superior oblique muscles

A–95
(G) V, trigeminal—chewing muscles

A–96
(C) VI, abducens—lateral rectus muscle

A–97
(A) VII, facial—tongue and facial muscles

A–98
(I) VIII, acoustic—hearing balance

A–99
(E) IX, glossopharyngeal—posterior pharynx

A–100
(J) X, vagus—taste to posterior tongue, diaphragm

A–101
(H) XI, accessory—trapezius muscles

A–102
(D) XII, hypoglossal—tongue

Questions

Q–103

On examining your patient, you discover an exaggerated thoracic concavity, or hunchback. This is known as

(A) normal.
(B) lordosis
(C) kyphosis
(D) scoliosis

Your Answer _____

_____

Q–104

Which of the following is NOT a component of scene size-up?

(A) Body substance isolation
(B) Location of all patients
(C) Mechanism of injury
(D) Physical examination

Your Answer _____

_____

Correct Answers

A–103

(C) Kyphosis is an exaggerated thoracic concavity, or hunchback. Lordosis is an exaggerated lumbar concavity, or swayback. Scoliosis is a lateral curvature.

A–104

(D) A scene size-up includes body substance isolation, scene safety, location of all patients, mechanism of injury, and nature of the illness.

Questions

You arrive on the scene of a domestic dispute. You still hear loud voices coming from the home. A person runs out of the house yelling, "She's not breathing!" You should

(A) enter the home and begin treatment
(B) wait for law enforcement to secure the scene
(C) ask the person running out of the house what is going on
(D) go some distance away and wait until they call you back

Your Answer _____

_____

You arrive on the scene of patient with a persistent cough. The patient states that the cough has been productive for purulent sputum. Which body substance isolation procedure would you take?

(A) Gloves
(B) Mask
(C) Eye protection
(D) All of the above

Your Answer _____

_____

Correct Answers

A–105

(B) The scene is not safe. You should not be close enough for the person running out of the house to come to your location. Even if you are close enough, you should wait until the scene has been deemed safe by law enforcement. Scene safety comes first.

A–106

(D) In this situation, you need to wear gloves, a mask, and eye protection to protect yourself. This patient is most likely suffering from a contagious respiratory infection (tuberculosis causes hemoptysis, night sweats, fatigue, etc.).

Questions

Q–107

Which of the following is the correct order of priorities for scene safety?

I. You
II. Your crew
III. Other responding personnel
IV. Your patient
V. Bystanders

(A) I, II, III, IV, V   (C) IV, I, III, II, V
(B) I, IV, II, III, V   (D) IV, II, III, I, V

Your Answer _____

Q–108

You arrive on the scene of a vehicle that went over an embankment. The driver is yelling that he is injured and his passenger is unresponsive. You are on a transportation unit with no rescue equipment. You should

(A) have your partner wait at the top of the embankment while you carefully climb down to the patients
(B) wait for a rescue unit to arrive with rescue equipment
(C) ask the patient if they can get out of the vehicle
(D) do none of the above

Your Answer _____

Correct Answers

A–107

(A) The correct order is you, your crew, other responding personnel, your patient, and bystanders.

A–108

(B) In this scenario, the best response is to wait until the rescue unit arrives with the appropriate equipment. You should never attempt a rescue that puts you or anyone else in grave danger. You cannot help anyone if you get injured.

Questions

Who directs the response and coordinates resources at the scene of a multicasualty incident (MCI)?

(A) Medical officer
(B) Paramedic
(C) Triage officer
(D) Incident commander

Your Answer _____

You are at the scene of an MCI. You have been assigned the role of triage officer. You should

(A) perform a triage assessment on every patient
(B) treat all priority-1 and priority-2 patients
(C) stabilize each patient before moving to the next patient
(D) do all the above

Your Answer _____

Correct Answers

A–109

(D) The incident commander is the person who directs the response and coordinates resources at the scene of an MCI. Each of the other people listed may assist and serve a specific role but does not direct the response and coordinate the resources in total.

A–110

(A) The triage officer can be the most difficult role to play. A triage officer should do a triage assessment on each patient and prioritize each patient for immediate or delayed response. The triage officer should not treat patients but rather triage patients until all patients have been accounted for.

Questions

Index of suspicion is

(A) the level of concern you have regarding scene safety
(B) your anticipation of possible injuries based on the mechanism of injury
(C) a term used by law enforcement to determine who is at fault in a motor vehicle accident
(D) part of the treatment for a trauma patient

Your Answer _____

911

You are treating a head injury patient. You notice her arms are flexed and her legs are extended. This is referred to as

(A) decerebrate
(B) decorticate
(C) lethargic
(D) postictal

Your Answer _____

Correct Answers

A–111

(B)   The index of suspicion is your anticipation of possible injuries based on the mechanism of injury. For example, if the steering wheel is deformed, you would have a high index of suspicion that the patient has chest injuries.

A–112

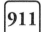

(B)   Decorticate is when a patient's arms are flexed and legs are extended. Decerebrate is when the patient's arms and legs are extended.

Questions

AVPU is used to describe a patient's mental status. The initials stand for

(A) alert, verbal, painful, unresponsive
(B) able, vortex, painful, unresponsive
(C) alert, verbal, positive, unopened
(D) ample, value, positive, unopened

Your Answer _____

An adult's normal range of pulse rate is

(A) 80–100
(B) 80–120
(C) 60–80
(D) 60–100

Your Answer _____

Correct Answers

A–113

(A) AVPU stands for alert, verbal, painful, unresponsive.

A–114

(D) An adult patient's normal heart rate is between 60 and 100.

Questions

Which of the following is NOT a feature of high-priority patients?

(A) Has poor general impression
(B) Went through a complicated childbirth
(C) Is responsive and follows commands
(D) Has uncontrolled bleeding

Your Answer _____

Which mechanism of injury is NOT a prediction of a serious internal injury for an adult?

(A) Fall from 15 feet
(B) Motorcycle crash
(C) Penetration of the head, chest, or abdomen
(D) Rollover of vehicle

Your Answer _____

Correct Answers

A–115

(C) Characteristics of high-priority patients include poor general impression, unresponsiveness, responsiveness but inability to follow commands, difficulty breathing, signs and symptoms of hypoperfusion, complicated childbirth, chest pain and blood pressure below 100 systolic, uncontrolled bleeding, severe pain, and multiple injuries.

A–116

(A) To be a prediction of a serious internal injury, the fall must be from higher than 20 feet.

Questions

You are examining your 28-year-old male patient. When you palpate the patient's chest, you notice subcutaneous emphysema. You would suspect this patient to have

(A) pink, frothy sputum
(B) cardiac tamponade
(C) pneumothorax
(D) fractured ribs

Your Answer _____

Which membrane covers the inner chest wall?

(A) Visceral pleura
(B) Parietal pleura
(C) Subarachnoid pleura
(D) Meninges

Your Answer _____

Correct Answers

A–117

(C) Although subcutaneous emphysema can be seen in the other listed conditions, it is primarily indicative of a pneumothorax.

A–118

(B) The parietal pleura is a thin membrane that covers the inner chest wall. The visceral pleura covers the lungs.

Questions

Q–119

Which of the following is a late sign of a tension pneumothorax?

(A) Hypotension
(B) Hypertension
(C) Tracheal deviation
(D) Unequal air movement

Your Answer _____

Q–120

911

You are treating a patient who was involved in an altercation. When you expose the chest, you notice a wound that appears to be caused by a knife. The wound is open, and you hear a sucking sound. The most appropriate treatment for this patient would be

(A) applying a Vaseline occlusive bandage
(B) applying a 4 × 4 and sealing three sides
(C) performing a chest decompression
(D) sticking your finger in the hole to check for depth of the wound

Your Answer _____

Correct Answers

A–119

(C) Tracheal deviation is a late sign of a tension pneumothorax. The trachea deviates as a result of air building up in the chest cavity and pushing the good lung away from the collapsed lung, thus deviating the trachea.

A–120

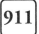

(A) The best treatment for a sucking chest injury is to seal the wound with a Vaseline gauze bandage. A 4×4 is porous and will not seal a sucking chest wound. There is no need to do a chest decompression because the patient is not suffering from a tension pneumothorax. You should not stick your finger in the wound.

Questions

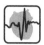

Which of the following is the classic sign or symptom of pulmonary edema?

(A) Chest pain
(B) Difficulty swallowing
(C) Pale, cool skin
(D) Pink, frothy sputum

Your Answer _____

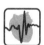

You check your patient for jugular vein distention. When you sit the patient at a 60-degree angle, you see distention. This may be a result of all the following EXCEPT

(A) cardiac tamponade
(B) hypovolemia
(C) tension pneumothorax
(D) right heart failure

Your Answer _____

Correct Answers

A–121

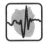

(D)   Pink, frothy sputum is a classic sign of pulmonary edema. The other signs and symptoms can also be seen in pulmonary edema but could be indicative of other conditions.

A–122

(B)   Hypovolemia is not a potential cause of jugular vein distention. Distention beyond 45 degrees is significant because it indicates that something is inhibiting blood return to the heart.

Questions

Your patient is suffering from congestive heart failure. When you listen to the patient's respiration, you are most likely to hear

(A) expiratory crackles
(B) stridor
(C) inspiratory crackles
(D) expiratory wheezing

Your Answer _____

Which sound would you expect to hear from a patient with chronic obstructive pulmonary disease?

(A) Expiratory crackles
(B) Stridor
(C) Inspiratory crackles
(D) Expiratory wheezes

Your Answer _____

Correct Answers

A–123

(C) Inspiratory crackles indicate either congestive heart failure or pulmonary edema.

A–124

(D) You would expect to hear expiratory wheezes in patients suffering from COPD or asthma as a result of bronchospasm.

Questions

Q–125

You are examining your patient's pulses. You notice that the patient has unequal pulses in the upper extremities. This finding suggests

(A) thoracic aneurysm
(B) abdominal aneurysm
(C) cerebral aneurysm
(D) none of the above

Your Answer _____

_____

Q–126

You are examining the patient's pupils and notice they are pinpoint. Which of the following is a possible cause?

(A) Anticholinergic drug overdose
(B) Hypovolemia
(C) Head injury
(D) Narcotic overdose

Your Answer _____

_____

Correct Answers

A–125

(A) If a patient has unequal pulses in the upper extremities, you would suspect a thoracic aneurysm. If the pulses are unequal in the lower extremities, you would suspect an abdominal aortic dissection.

A–126

(D) Pinpoint pupils often indicate a narcotic overdose. Anticholinergic drug overdose usually results in dilated pupils. Head injuries usually are indicated by unequal-sized pupils. With hypovolemia, the pupils are usually slow to react but eventually dilate.

Questions

You are treating your patient and she begins to vomit a coffee-ground emesis. You would suspect

(A) upper GI tract bleeding
(B) lower GI tract bleeding
(C) that the patient ate coffee grounds
(D) a ruptured liver

Your Answer _____

PSAP stands for

(A) pulse, sensation, alteration, pupils
(B) Public Safety Answering Point
(C) pulsating, sensation, aptitude, preference
(D) Preferred Standard Algorithm Protocol

Your Answer _____

Correct Answers

A–127

(A) Coffee-ground emesis is a result of the blood mixing with stomach acids and suggests an upper GI tract bleed.

A–128

(B) PSAP stands for Public Safety Answering Point. This is typically where 911 calls are answered.

Questions

911

Which communication system allows for two-way communications?

(A) Simplex
(B) Duplex
(C) Monoplex
(D) Miniplex

Your Answer _____

911

Which of the following is NOT an element of good documentation?

(A) Accuracy
(B) Legibility
(C) Absence of pertinent negatives
(D) Timeliness

Your Answer _____

Correct Answers

A–129

911

(B) A duplex system allows for two-way communications. A simplex system allows for one-way communication.

A–130

911

(C) The elements of good documentation are accuracy, legibility, timeliness, absence of alterations, and professionalism.

Questions

The trachea divides into the right and left mainstem bronchi at the

(A) carina
(B) larynx
(C) alveoli
(D) glottic opening

Your Answer _____

Exchange of oxygen and carbon dioxide takes place in the

(A) bronchioles
(B) bronchus
(C) bronchi
(D) alveoli

Your Answer _____

Correct Answers

A–131

(A) The trachea divides into the right and left mainstem bronchi at the carina.

A–132

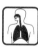

(D) The exchange of oxygen and carbon dioxide takes place in the alveoli.

Questions

Which of the following is NOT a part of the gas exchange process in the lungs?

(A) Inhalation
(B) Ventilation
(C) Diffusion
(D) Perfusion

Your Answer _____

What part of the brain controls ventilation?

(A) Cerebellum
(B) Medulla
(C) Frontal lobe
(D) Pons delta

Your Answer _____

Correct Answers

(A) Inhalation is part of ventilation (the other part is exhalation). Ventilation, diffusion, and perfusion are parts of the gas exchange process.

(B) The medulla is located at the lower portion of the brainstem. It controls ventilation.

Questions

What is the normal total lung capacity of a male?

(A) 500 mL
(B) 1,000 L
(C) 6,000 L
(D) 6,000 mL

Your Answer _____

In a COPD patient, the Pco_2 is chronically elevated, forcing the body to rely on

(A) Po_2 to regulate respirations
(B) CO_2 to regulate respirations
(C) pH to regulate respirations
(D) none of the above

Your Answer _____

Correct Answers

A–135

(D) The total lung capacity of a normal male is 6,000 mL.

A–136

(A) P_{O_2} regulates respirations in patients with COPD, a condition that causes P_{CO_2} to be chronically elevated.

Questions

Which condition is NOT necessary for lung perfusion?

(A) Adequate blood flow
(B) Normal blood pressure
(C) Intact pulmonary capillaries
(D) Efficient pumping of blood by the heart

Your Answer _____

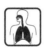

You are treating a 69-year-old male whom you suspect has chronic bronchitis. He states that he smokes two to three packs of cigarettes a day. He has shortness of breath, has been coughing a thick mucous, and is dehydrated. The best treatment for this patient would include

(A) oxygen, IV, and corticosteroids
(B) oxygen, IV fluids at TKO rate, and corticosteroids
(C) oxygen, fluid challenge via IV, and corticosteroids
(D) none of the above

Your Answer _____

Correct Answers

A–137

(B) Normal blood pressure is not necessary for lung perfusion.

A–138

(C) Because the patient is dehydrated, you should give a fluid bolus. In addition, he will likely need a corticosteroid.

Questions

Which of the following is NOT a trigger or inducer of asthma?

(A) Warm air
(B) Exercise
(C) Irritants
(D) Stress

Your Answer _____

At which phase in an asthma attack is histamine released?

(A) Phase 1
(B) Phase 2
(C) Phase 3
(D) Phase 4

Your Answer _____

Correct Answers

A–139

(A) The triggers or inducers of asthma are cold air, exercise, irritants, stress, environmental allergens, foods, and certain medications.

A–140

(A) There are two phases to an asthma attack. In phase 1, a chemical mediator is released called histamine.

Questions

You are treating a patient who has severe shortness of breath. When you auscultate breath sounds, you hear diminished breath sounds but no wheezing. The patient's chest is distended, and the patient appears to be exhausted. You would suspect

(A) COPD
(B) status asthmaticus
(C) CHF
(D) pneumonia

Your Answer _____

Which of the following is (are) used to determine if a patient has pneumonia?

(A) Physical examination
(B) X-ray findings
(C) Blood cultures
(D) All of the above

Your Answer _____

Correct Answers

A–141

(B) Just because a patient has no wheezing does not mean that he or she is not having an asthma attack. In this situation, the patient is in the advanced stages of an asthma attack. You should prepare for the patient going into respiratory arrest.

A–142

(D) Diagnosing pneumonia in the field is difficult because it requires performing a physical examination, viewing x-ray findings, and reviewing laboratory cultures.

Questions

How much greater is carbon monoxide's affinity for hemoglobin than oxygen's affinity for hemoglobin?

(A) 100 times
(B) 200 times
(C) 300 times
(D) 400 times

Your Answer _____

Your patient is complaining of headache. She has been nauseated and is vomiting. She appears to be agitated and is confused. She states that she has been having chest pain and does not have good coordination. You would suspect that this patient is suffering from

(A) myocardial infarction
(B) COPD
(C) stroke
(D) carbon monoxide poisoning

Your Answer _____

Correct Answers

(B) Carbon monoxide has an affinity for hemoglobin that is 200 times that of oxygen.

(D) This patient is exhibiting the signs and symptoms of carbon monoxide poisoning. Such a patient can escalate to seizures and then death.

Questions

Your patient is having trouble breathing. She explains that it came on suddenly. She is 22 years old and has no medical problems. She states that the only medication she takes is birth control pills. She has no known allergies and is otherwise in good health. When you conduct your examination, you find breath sounds diminished on her left side. Her blood pressure is 100/60 and pulse is 100. You notice she has jugular venous distention (JVD). You would suspect

(A) pulmonary contusion
(B) pneumonia
(C) pulmonary embolism
(D) asthma

Your Answer _____

_____

Fast Fact

EMT management salaries are generally below $50,000.

Correct Answers

A–145

(C) The signs and symptoms in this patient are suggestive of a pulmonary embolism, which is common in women taking birth control pills.

Career Pulse

The NREMT examinations are developed so that they measure the important aspects of pre-hospital care practice.

Questions

You are called to assist a 24-year-old male who is having trouble breathing. The patient is tall and very slender. He complains of a sharp, pleuritic chest pain, and you notice decreased breath sounds on the right side. You would suspect

(A) spontaneous pneumothorax
(B) pneumonia
(C) pulmonary embolism
(D) none of the above

Your Answer _____

Cardiac output is defined as
(A) Tidal volume × Heart rate
(B) Tidal volume × Stroke volume
(C) Stroke volume × Heart rate
(D) Blood pressure × Stroke volume

Your Answer _____

Correct Answers

A–146

(A) Individuals who are tall and slender are at higher risk for spontaneous pneumothorax. These patients tend to be 20 to 40 years of age and typically are smokers.

A–147

(C) Cardiac output is calculated by multiplying stroke volume by heart rate.

Questions

Match each of the following terms to the correct number of beats.

Q–148 SA node

Q–149 AV node

Q–150 Purkinje system

(A) 15–40 beats per minute
(B) 15–40 beats per second
(C) 40–60 beats per second
(D) 40–60 beats per minute
(E) 60–100 beats per minute
(F) 60–100 beats per second

Your Answer _____

_____

Career Pulse

Test items for the NREMT exams are developed in relation to tasks identified in the practice analysis.

Correct Answers

A–148 to 150

A–148
(E) SA node—60–100 beats per minute

A–149
(D) AV node—40–60 beats per minute

A–150
(A) Purkinje system—15–40 beats per minute

Fast Fact *Because paid firefighters are unionized, their salaries tend to be higher and their jobs coveted in some areas.*

Questions

The term describing the propagation of an electrical impulse from one cell to another is

(A) excitability
(B) conductivity
(C) automaticity
(D) contractility

Your Answer _____

_____

Which of the following is NOT a common cause of artifact on EKGs?

(A) Muscle tremors
(B) Lead placement
(C) Patient movement
(D) Machine malfunction

Your Answer _____

_____

Correct Answers

A–151

(B) Conductivity refers to the propagation of an electrical impulse from one cell to another.

A–152

(B) Lead placement does not typically cause artifact on EKGs. Muscle tremors, shivering, patient movement, loose electrodes, 60-hertz interference, and machine malfunction are common causes of artifact.

Questions

Match each of the following leads to the correct position of the heart examined.

Q–153 I and aVL

Q–154 II, III, and aVF

Q–155 aVR

Q–156 V1 and V2

Q–157 V3 and V4

Q–158 V5 and V6

(A) Right ventricle and anterior portions of heart
(B) Anterior and lateral walls of left ventricle
(C) Left side of heart in vertical plane
(D) Intraventricular septum and anterior wall of left ventricle
(E) Inferior side of heart
(F) Right side of heart in vertical plane

Your Answer _____

_____

Fast Fact

Volunteers in general are not paid but some receive nominal monies for their services and some are able to earn pensions.

Correct Answers

A–153 to 158

A–153

(C) I and aVL—left side of heart in vertical plane

A–154

(E) II, III, and aVF—inferior side of heart

A–155

(F) aVR—right side of heart in vertical plane

A–156

(A) V1 and V2—right ventricle and anterior portions of heart

A–157

(D) V3 and V4—intraventricular septum and anterior wall of left ventricle

A–158

(B) V5 and V6—anterior and lateral walls of left ventricle.

Questions

Q–159

Which sequence does a myocardial infarction typically follow?

(A) Ischemia, necrosis, injury
(B) Injury, necrosis, ischemia
(C) Necrosis, injury, ischemia
(D) Ischemia, injury, necrosis

Your Answer _____

Q–160

Sinus bradycardia results from

(A) slowing of the AV node
(B) slowing of the SA node
(C) increased sympathetic tone
(D) right bundle branch block

Your Answer _____

Correct Answers

A-159

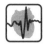

(D) Ischemia is typically followed by injury and then necrosis in myocardial infarctions.

A-160

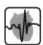

(B) Sinus bradycardia results from slowing of the SA node. One of the conditions that may cause this is increased parasympathetic tone.

Questions

You arrive on the scene and find your patient sitting on a chair with no real complaints at this time other than feeling a little weak. He has no significant medical problems. His blood pressure is 120/80, and he is not in acute distress. You attach the EKG monitor and receive the reading shown in Figure 1. You determine that the patient's rhythm is

(A) normal sinus rhythm
(B) second-degree AV block type 2
(C) sinus bradycardia
(D) third-degree AV block

Your Answer _____

_____

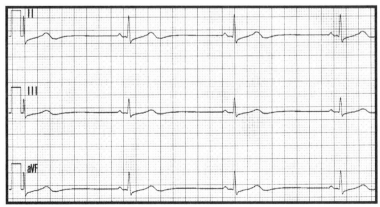

Figure 1

Correct Answers

A–161

(C) This patient's rhythm is sinus bradycardia.

Career Pulse

Paramedic education programs are encouraged to review the NREMT Practice Analysis when teaching courses and when performing final reviews of student's abilities to deliver the tasks necessary for competent patient practice.

Questions

Which of the following is the appropriate treatment for the patient described in *question 161*?

(A) Oxygen, IV, atropine 5 mg
(B) Oxygen, IV, monitor
(C) Oxygen, IV, pacer
(D) Oxygen, IV, dopamine drip

Your Answer _____

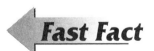

Most EMS workers across the United States are volunteers.

Correct Answers

(B) Since the patient is not in any distress, you would monitor the patient and treat any significant changes.

Career Pulse

Individual examination items are developed by members of the EMS community serving on item writing committees convened by the NREMT.

Questions

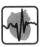

You are treating a patient involved in a motor vehicle accident. She appears to have multiple injuries. You attach the EKG monitor and receive the reading shown in Figure 2. What is the patient's rhythm?

(A) Sinus tachycardia
(B) Ventricular tachycardia
(C) Atrial fibrillation
(D) Paroxysmal supraventricular tachycardia

Your Answer _____

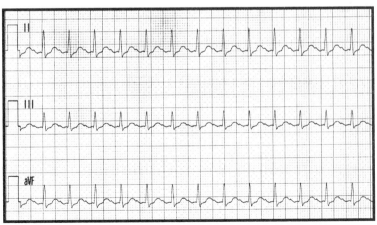

Figure 2

Correct Answers

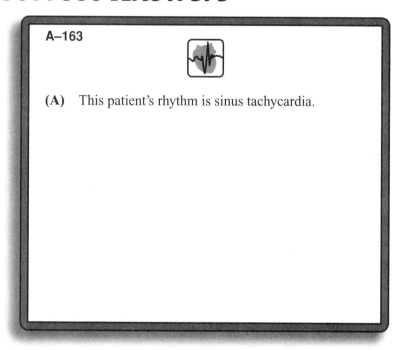

A–163

(A) This patient's rhythm is sinus tachycardia.

Fast Fact
EMTs administer first-aid treatment and life-support care to sick or injured persons in the prehospital setting.

Questions

Your patient tells you he feels like he is having palpitations. You attach the EKG monitor and receive the reading shown in Figure 3. You determine that the patient's rhythm is

(A) ventricular fibrillation
(B) ventricular tachycardia
(C) supraventricular tachycardia
(D) sinus tachycardia

Your Answer _____

_____

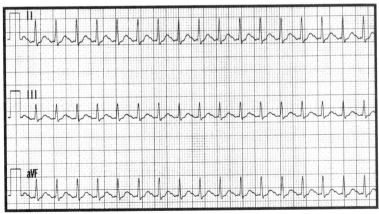

Figure 3

Correct Answers

A–164

(C) This patient's rhythm is supraventricular tachycardia. It is usually sudden in onset, may last minutes to hours, and terminates abruptly. Stress, overexertion, smoking, or ingestion of caffeine can precipitate supraventricular tachycardia.

Career Pulse

Items for the NREMT exams are reviewed for reading level and to ensure that no bias exists related to race, gender or ethnicity.

Questions

Your patient is having chest pain and difficulty breathing. She appears to be lethargic, and her blood pressure is 90/40. You attach the EKG monitor and receive the reading shown in Figure 4. You determine that the patient's rhythm is

(A) atrial flutter
(B) atrial fibrillation
(C) supraventricular tachycardia
(D) sinus tachycardia

Your Answer _____

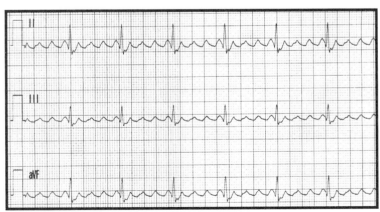

Figure 4

Correct Answers

A–165

(A) As shown in the figure, the P waves have been replaced by a sawtooth pattern, indicating that this patient is in atrial flutter. The atrial rate is somewhere in the range of 250 to 350 beats per minute. The ventricular rate varies with the ratio of AV conduction.

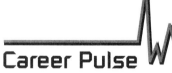

Career Pulse

Pilot items for the NREMT exams are administered to candidates during computer-adaptive exams. They are indistinguishable from scored items; however, they do not count for or against the candidate.

Questions

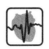

The heart rate of the patient described in *question 165* increases to 160 beats per minute. The treatment for the patient is

(A) oxygen, IV, atropine
(B) oxygen, IV, synchronized monophasic countershock of 100 joules
(C) oxygen, IV, unsynchronized monophasic counter-shock of 100 joules
(D) oxygen, IV, Cardizem

Your Answer _____

Fast Fact

EMTs operate equipment such as electrocardiograms (EKGs), external defibrillators and bag-valve mask resuscitators in advanced life-support environments.

Correct Answers

A–166

(B) This patient is unstable. She is exhibiting chest pain and shortness of breath, and she is hypotensive. In this situation, after administration of oxygen and an IV, a synchronized monophasic countershock of 100 joules is the most appropriate course of treatment. You may want to consider mild sedation before shocking.

Fast Fact *Paramedics assess the nature and extent of illness or injury to establish and prioritize medical procedures.*

Questions

Your patient tells you she is having trouble breathing and some chest pain. She is in her late sixties. Her pulse is tachycardic and hypotensive. She is sitting on the edge of her chair, and you notice she has positive JVD. You would suspect that this patient is suffering from

(A) myocardial infarction
(B) COPD
(C) CHF
(D) pneumonia

Your Answer _____

_____

 Fast Fact

Paramedics maintain vehicles, medical and communication equipment, first-aid equipment, and supplies.

Correct Answers

A–167

(C) This patient has the signs and symptoms of congestive heart failure.

Career Pulse

The NREMT Board of Directors determines the pass/fail score of the examination as guided by psychometric consultants.

Questions

You attach the EKG monitor to the patient described in *question 167* and receive the reading shown in Figure 5. You determine that the patient's rhythm is

(A) atrial flutter
(B) sinus tachycardia
(C) atrial tachycardia
(D) atrial fibrillation

Your Answer _____

_____

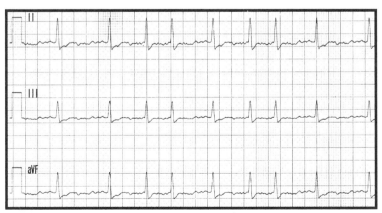

Figure 5

Correct Answers

A–168

(D)   Atrial fibrillation is classified by no discernible P waves, an irregular rhythm, and a tachycardic rate.

Fast Fact *Paramedics observe, record, and report to the physician the patient's condition or injury, the treatment provided, and the response to drugs and treatment.*

Questions

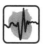

You are called to the home of a 59-year-old male who is complaining of flu-like symptoms. He has no significant medical problems. However, he states that he had some type of EKG abnormality but does not remember the name. You attach the EKG monitor and receive the reading shown in Figure 6. You determine that the patient's rhythm is

(A) Wenckebach
(B) first-degree AV block
(C) second-degree AV block type 2
(D) third-degree AV block

Your Answer _____

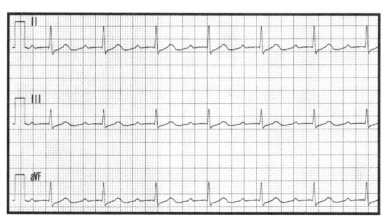

Figure 6

Correct Answers

(B) The rhythm is first-degree AV block. A first-degree AV block is characterized by a prolonged P-R interval. The other traits of the rhythm shown in the figure are typically normal.

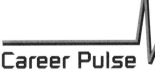

Career Pulse

The items and statistical data for the NREMT exams are reviewed by the National Registry to assure that each item and the examination are functioning properly. Statistics for the NREMT exams are generated for training sites, states, and/or national results.

Questions

What treatment should you provide for the patient described in *question 169*?

(A) Oxygen, IV, monitor patient
(B) Oxygen, IV, atropine
(C) Oxygen, IV, nitroglycerin
(D) No treatment is necessary

Your Answer _____

_____

Fast Fact

Paramedics perform emergency diagnostic and treatment procedures, such as stomach suction, airway management, and heart monitoring, during the ambulance ride.

Correct Answers

A–170

(A) This patient appears to have the "flu." Therefore, oxygen and IV are the only treatments that may be warranted at this time. First-degree AV block typically does not require any intervention.

Fast Fact *Paramedics administer drugs, orally or by injection, and perform intravenous procedures under a physician's direction.*

Questions

The rhythm shown in Figure 7 is

(A) first-degree AV block
(B) second-degree AV block type 1
(C) second-degree AV block type 2
(D) third-degree AV block

Your Answer _____

_____

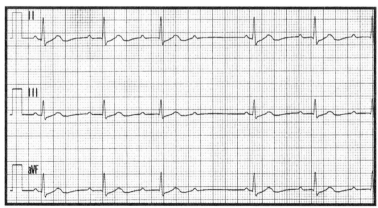

Figure 7

Correct Answers

A–171

(B) Second-degree AV block type 1, also known as Wenckebach, is characterized by an increasingly long P-R interval until a QRS complex is dropped.

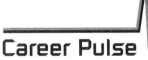

Career Pulse

All items for the NREMT exams have one correct or best answer as agreed upon by the Item Writing Committee. All items for the NREMT exams are multiple-choice items.

Questions

You arrive on the scene of a woman who has collapsed. You assess the patient and find she is pulseless and apneic. You attach the EKG monitor and receive the reading shown in Figure 8. You determine that the patient's rhythm is

(A) fine ventricular fibrillation
(B) ventricular fibrillation
(C) asystole
(D) torsades de pointes

Your Answer _____

_____

Figure 8

Correct Answers

A–172

(C) This patient is in asystole, which is characterized by an essentially flat line with no organized electrical activity.

Fast Fact Paramedics communicate with dispatchers and treatment center personnel to provide information about the situation, to arrange reception of victims, and to receive instructions for further treatment.

Questions

You begin CPR on the patient described in *question 172*. Which medication would you consider for this patient?

(A) Lidocaine
(B) Amiodarone
(C) Magnesium
(D) Epinephrine

Your Answer _____

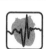

What would be the correct dosage of vasopressin for the patient described in *questions 172 and 173*?

(A) 40 units
(B) 1.5 mg/kg
(C) 300 mg
(D) 1 g

Your Answer _____

Correct Answers

A–173

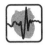

(D) You would give this patient epinephrine. Alternatively, you could give her vasopressin.

A–174

(A) The correct dosage of vasopressin would be 40 units IV or IO.

Questions

Your patient is unresponsive. You assess for breathing and pulses and cannot find any breathing or pulses. You attach the EKG monitor and receive the reading shown in Figure 9. You determine that the patient's rhythm is

(A) normal sinus rhythm
(B) pulseless electrical activity
(C) sinus bradycardia
(D) sinus tachycardia

Your Answer _____

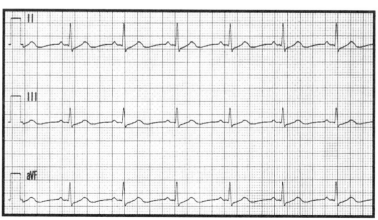

Figure 9

Correct Answers

A–175

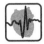

(A) The monitor shows a normal sinus rhythm. The algorithm you would follow is pulseless electrical activity (PEA), which is not a rhythm but rather is a term used to identify any rhythm that has organized electrical activity but does not have a pulse.

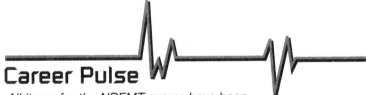

Career Pulse

All items for the NREMT exams have been reviewed for reading level and to also prevent regional bias.

Questions

Which of the following is NOT a potential contributing factor for PEA?

(A) Hypovolemia
(B) Hyperglycemia
(C) Hypothermia
(D) Hypoxia

Your Answer _____

_____

Which of the following is NOT typically a potential contributing factor for PEA?

(A) Tachypnea
(B) Toxins
(C) Tamponade
(D) Trauma

Your Answer _____

_____

Correct Answers

A–176

(B) The "six H's" that are possible contributing factors for PEA are hypovolemia, hypothermia, hypoxia, hydrogen ion or acidosis, hypokalemia or hyperkalemia, and hypoglycemia.

A–177

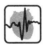

(A) The "five T's" that are possible contributing factors for PEA are toxins, tamponade, trauma, tension pneumothorax, and thrombosis.

Questions

You arrive on the scene to find a 62-year-old male complaining of chest pain. He is ashen in color and diaphoretic. His pulse is about 48, and his blood pressure is 88/40. You attach the EKG monitor and receive the reading shown in Figure 10. You determine that the patient's rhythm is

(A) first-degree AV block
(B) second-degree AV block type 1
(C) second-degree AV block type 2
(D) third-degree AV block

Your Answer _____

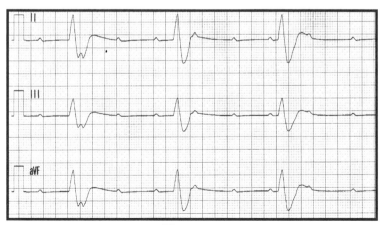

Figure 10

Correct Answers

(D)   This patient is in third-degree AV block. The P waves and the QRS complexes are marching to a different beat; that is, there is no relationship between them.

Career Pulse

All items for the NREMT exams have been reviewed to ensure they cover current clinical therapy. They relate to the practice of out-of-hospital care, and when not in a practice case, the scenarios have answers that are available in common EMS textbooks.

Questions

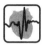

The treatment for the patient described in *question 178* would include

(A) oxygen, IV, synchronized monophasic countershock of 50 joules
(B) oxygen, IV, pacer
(C) oxygen, IV 0.5 mg atropine
(D) oxygen, IV, 1 mg/kg of lidocaine, pacer

Your Answer _____

_____

Fast Fact

Paramedics coordinate work with other emergency medical team members, and police and fire department personnel.

Correct Answers

A–179

(B) Oxygen, IV, and a pacer is the preferred treatment. Remember, do not give lidocaine to a patient whose underlying rhythm is bradycardic.

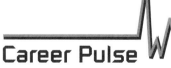

Career Pulse

The NREMT exam is constructed so that anybody taking the exam that can meet the standard can pass. The purpose of the NREMT exam is not to identify the best, but to identify who is "competent."

Questions

Your patient is complaining of trouble breathing. She has some mild chest tightness. You attach the EKG monitor and receive the reading shown in Figure 11. You determine that the patient's rhythm is

(A) supraventricular tachycardia
(B) third-degree AV block
(C) normal sinus rhythm with premature ventricular contractions (PVCs)
(D) atrial flutter

Your Answer _____

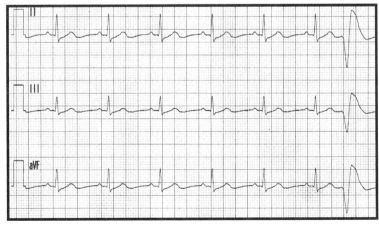

Figure 11

Correct Answers

A–180

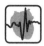

(C) This patient has a normal sinus rhythm with premature ventricular contractions. The shortness of breath could be the underlying reason for the PVCs.

Career Pulse

Criterion-based examinations like the National Registry have only one score that counts: that the candidate either meets the criteria (passes) or does not meet the criteria (fails).

Questions

For the patient described in *question 180*, the first line of treatment for the PVCs is

(A) lidocaine 1 mg/kg
(B) oxygen
(C) amiodarone 300 mg
(D) lidocaine 1.5 mg/kg

Your Answer _____

Career Pulse

A score of 85% on the NREMT examination is not a "B," or "good job." NREMT doesn't measure achievement, but rather measures if the candidate meets the criteria of entry-level competency.

Correct Answers

A–181

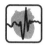

(B) The first line of treatment for this patient is oxygen. This patient is having shortness of breath, and the oxygen may reduce or eliminate the PVCs. No specific treatment is needed for PVCs.

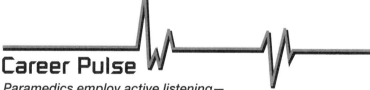

Career Pulse

Paramedics employ active listening— giving full attention to what other people are saying, taking time to understand the points being made, asking questions as appropriate, and not interrupting at inappropriate times.

Questions

The rhythm shown in Figure 12 is

(A) supraventricular tachycardia
(B) ventricular fibrillation
(C) ventricular tachycardia
(D) atrial fibrillation

Your Answer _____

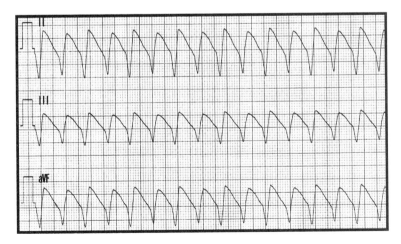

Figure 12

Correct Answers

A–182

(C) The rhythm shown in the figure is ventricular tachy-cardia.

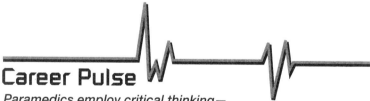

Career Pulse

Paramedics employ critical thinking— using logic and reasoning to identify the strengths and weaknesses of alternative solutions, conclusions or approaches to problems.

Questions

At which of the following rates of dopamine infusion would the beta-receptors be more affected than the alpha-receptors?

(A) 1–2 mg/kg/min
(B) 2–10 mcg/kg/min
(C) 10–15 mcg/kg/min
(D) 15–20 mcg/kg/min

Your Answer _____

You arrive on the scene of a 22-year-old patient who states that she has been bleeding from her vagina. She says that the flow has been very heavy and that she is lightheaded. Which of the following is the correct treatment?

(A) Apply oxygen, start an IV, apply an absorbing pad, transport
(B) Apply oxygen, start an IV, have patient cross legs to apply pressure, transport
(C) Apply oxygen, start an IV, pack the vagina with absorbing pads, transport
(D) None of the above

Your Answer _____

Correct Answers

A–183

(B) At 2–10 mcg/kg/min, dopamine primarily affects the beta-receptors. At 10–15 mcg/kg/min, it affects both alpha- and beta-receptors; and at 15–20 mcg/kg/min, it primarily affects alpha-receptors.

A–184

(A) The appropriate treatment for this patient is to apply oxygen, start an IV for fluid replacement, apply an absorbing pad, and transport to the hospital. Packing the vagina is not appropriate because you should never insert anything in the vagina.

Questions

Your patient is complaining of palpitations in her chest. She has never experienced anything like it before. Her pulse is about 90. You attach the EKG monitor, and it is showing supraventricular tachycardia, as shown in Figure 13. You apply high-flow oxygen and start an IV. You should consider administering

(A) nothing, but monitor the patient
(B) adenosine 6 mg IVP
(C) countershock of 50 joules
(D) nitroglycerin sublingual

Your Answer _____

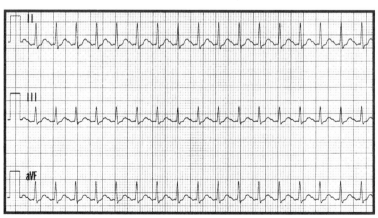

Figure 13

Correct Answers

A–185

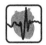

(B) In this situation, you want to reduce the patient's rate heart. The fact that her pulse and EKG rate do not match indicates that she is not perfusing with every beat. The best choice for this patient is to administer 6 mg of adenosine IVP.

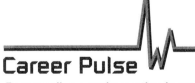

Career Pulse

Paramedics employ active learning —
understanding the implications of new information for both
current and future problem solving and decision-making.

Questions

Your patient is a 20-year-old female complaining of abdominal pain. She states that her pain radiates to her left shoulder. She has tenderness over the left side of her abdomen. She does not know if she is pregnant, but her period is late. You would suspect

(A) ruptured liver
(B) ruptured spleen
(C) ectopic pregnancy
(D) abdominal aneurysm

Your Answer _____

You are preparing your trauma patient for transport. She is 28 years old and is 7 months pregnant. The proper position for this patient is

(A) tilted to the right side
(B) tilted to the left side
(C) a normal supine position
(D) the Trendelenberg position

Your Answer _____

Correct Answers

A–186

(C) This patient's presentation suggests ectopic pregnancy.

A–187

(B) You should transport this patient tilted to her left side. This will help minimize supine hypotension owing to inferior vena cava compression caused by the gravid uterus.

Questions

Spontaneous abortions typically occur

(A) before the 20th week of pregnancy
(B) before the 16th week of pregnancy
(C) before the 12th week of pregnancy
(D) before the 8th week of pregnancy

Your Answer _____

Which of the following is NOT a predisposing factor of abruptio placentae?

(A) Multiparity
(B) Maternal hypotension
(C) Trauma
(D) Cocaine use

Your Answer _____

Correct Answers

A–188

(C) Spontaneous abortions typically occur before the 12th week of pregnancy.

A–189

(B) The predisposing factors of abruptio placentae are multiparity, maternal hypertension, trauma, cocaine use, increasing maternal age, and a history of abruption with a previous pregnancy.

Questions

The following scenario applies to questions 190–192.

As you gather the information on your pregnant patient, she tells you she is nine months along, and that her doctor said something about her placenta blocking her cervical opening.

Q–190

You would suspect

(A) a breach baby
(B) placenta previa
(C) abruptio placentae
(D) miscarriage

Your Answer _____

_____

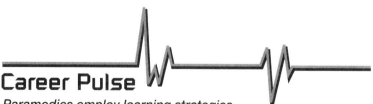

Career Pulse

*Paramedics employ learning strategies—
selecting and using training/instructional methods and
procedures appropriate for the situation when learning
or teaching new things.*

Correct Answers

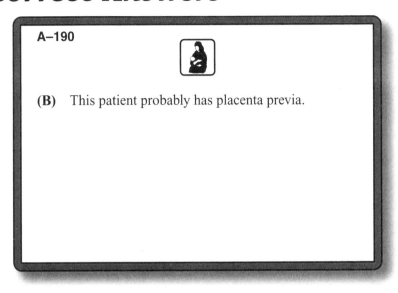

A–190

(B) This patient probably has placenta previa.

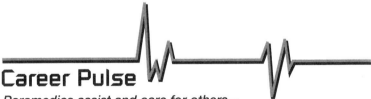

Career Pulse

*Paramedics assist and care for others—
providing personal assistance, medical attention, emotional
support, or other personal care to others such as coworkers,
customers, or patients.*

Questions

Which of the following is the greatest potential threat for the patient?

(A) Uncontrolled bleeding
(B) Placenta rupturing
(C) Miscarriage
(D) Severe pain

Your Answer _____

_____

Which of the following is the best treatment for this patient?

(A) IV
(B) Prepare for delivery
(C) Place pressure on the vagina to prevent delivery
(D) Immediate transport to the hospital

Your Answer _____

_____

Correct Answers

A–191

(A) The greatest threat for this patient is uncontrolled bleeding. A patient who is diagnosed with this condition typically is placed on bed rest.

A–192

(D) This patient should be transported to the hospital immediately. An IV can be started on the way, and you should prepare for a delivery, but this patient will most likely need a cesarean section.

Questions

Q–193

Which of the following is the classic sign of central abruptio placentae?

(A) Sudden sharp, tearing pain
(B) Massive hemorrhaging
(C) No pain
(D) All of the above

Your Answer _____

Q–194

Braxton-Hicks contractions are

(A) false labor
(B) a sign that the baby is ready to deliver
(C) a sign of possible miscarriage
(D) none of the above

Your Answer _____

Correct Answers

A–193

(A) The classic sign of central abruptio placentae is a sudden sharp, tearing pain. The abdomen may also become boardlike on palpation. Central is one of the two types of partial abruptio placentae. The other type is marginal, which is characterized by vaginal bleeding with no increase in pain. A complete abruptio placentae is characterized by massive vaginal bleeding and profound maternal hypotension.

A–194

(A) Braxton-Hicks contractions are false labor.

Questions

The following scenario applies to questions 195–197.

Your patient is a 34-year-old female who is 8 months pregnant. She is complaining of a headache and says she has visual disturbances. You notice she has a lot of edema. Her blood pressure is 188/110.

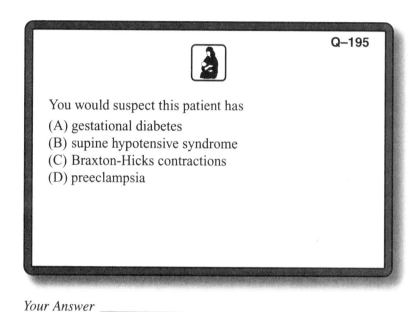

Q–195

You would suspect this patient has

(A) gestational diabetes
(B) supine hypotensive syndrome
(C) Braxton-Hicks contractions
(D) preeclampsia

Your Answer _____

Correct Answers

(D) This patient's signs and symptoms are classic for preeclampsia.

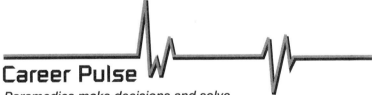

Career Pulse

Paramedics make decisions and solve problems by analyzing information and evaluating results.

Questions

Which of the following is the most appropriate treatment for this patient?

(A) Dim the lights
(B) Transport quickly without lights and siren
(C) Keep the patient calm
(D) All of the above

Your Answer _____

_____

Your patient in the above situation begins to seize. The most appropriate treatment would be to administer

(A) Valium
(B) Dilantin
(C) magnesium sulfate
(D) no medications

Your Answer _____

_____

Correct Answers

A–196

(D) Preeclampsia can be a life-threatening condition. You would keep the patient calm, dim the lights, and transport quickly without the lights and siren. You would not want to do anything to get this patient excited.

A–197

(C) In this situation, the best therapy would be magnesium sulfate intravenously.

Questions

Match each of the following stages of labor to the correct definition.

Q–198 Stage 1

Q–199 Stage 2

Q–200 Stage 3

(A) Expulsion (C) Contractual
(B) Placental   (D) Dilation

Your Answer _____

_____

Q–201

911

Kinetic energy is equal to

(A) Mass × Velocity
(B) (Mass × Velocity^2) / 2
(C) Mass × Weight
(D) Velocity × Mass^2 / 2

Your Answer _____

_____

Correct Answers

A–198 to 200

A–198

(D) The first stage of labor is dilation. This stage is characterized by dilation of the cervix to 10 cm in preparation for delivery of the infant.

A–199

(A) Expulsion is the second stage in labor. This stage is characterized by delivery of the infant.

A–200

(B) The third stage of labor is the placental stage. This stage is characterized by the delivery of the placenta, or afterbirth.

A–201

(B) Kinetic energy is equal to the mass or weight multiplied by the velocity or speed squared; this total is then divided by 2. Kinetic energy is the energy produced by the motion of an object having mass.

Questions

911

Which of the following injuries account for the majority of motor vehicle fatalities?

(A) Head injuries
(B) Internal injuries: chest, abdomen, or pelvis
(C) Spinal and chest fractures
(D) Extremity fractures

Your Answer _____

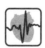

Which of the following is NOT one of the four elements that affect stroke volume?

(A) Preload
(B) Afterload
(C) Ventricular filling
(D) Ventricular discharge

Your Answer _____

Correct Answers

A–202

911

(A) The incidence of fatalities by injuries are head injuries, 47.7%; internal injuries, 37.3%; spinal and chest fractures, 8.3%; fractures to the extremities, 2.0%.

A–203

(D) The four elements that affect stroke volume are preload, afterload, ventricular filling, and cardiac contractility.

Questions

Which of the following systems slows the heart rate?

(A) Parasympathetic nervous system
(B) Sympathetic nervous system
(C) Parasympathetic cardiovascular system
(D) Sympathetic cardiovascular system

Your Answer _____

The Frank-Starling mechanism

(A) increases cardiac output
(B) increases cardiac contractility
(C) decreases cardiac output
(D) decreases cardiac contractility

Your Answer _____

Correct Answers

A–204

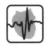

(A) The parasympathetic nervous system slows the heart rate, and the sympathetic nervous system, through the action of hormones, increases it.

A–205

(B) The Frank-Starling mechanism results in an increase in cardiac contractility because of increased myocardial muscle stretching that leads to an increase in stroke volume.

Questions

A patient has melena. This is defined as

(A) skin cancer
(B) black tarlike feces
(C) vomiting blood
(D) none of the above

Your Answer _____

A fractured pelvis can result in a blood loss of

(A) 500 mL
(B) 750 mL
(C) 1,500 mL
(D) 2,000 mL

Your Answer _____

Correct Answers

A–206

(B) Melena is black tarlike feces caused by gastrointestinal bleeding. Melanoma is a type of skin cancer. Hematemesis is vomiting blood.

A–207

(D) A fractured pelvis can result in a blood loss of up to 2,000 mL. A fractured femur can cause up to 1,500 mL of blood loss; a fractured tibia or humerus, up to 750 mL; and a large contusion, up to 500 mL.

Questions

911

You are assessing your patient. The patient states that he becomes dizzy whenever he stands up. You perform a tilt test. If the patient has relative hypovolemia, you would expect to find

(A) a drop in blood pressure of 20 mm Hg
(B) a decrease in pulse rate of 20 beats per minute
(C) both A and B
(D) neither A nor B

Your Answer _____

_____

911

You discover an open neck wound on your patient. You should

(A) apply a dry sterile dressing
(B) apply an occlusive dressing
(C) apply a bulky dressing
(D) let the wound remain open

Your Answer _____

_____

Correct Answers

A–208

911

(A)   You would expect to find that a drop in blood pressure of 20 mm Hg or an increase in the pulse rate of 10 beats per minute.

A–209

911

(B)   You should cover any open neck wound with an occlusive dressing held firmly in place.

Questions

911

A state of inadequate tissue perfusion is called

(A) shock
(B) hypovolemia
(C) cyanosis
(D) cardiac insufficiency

Your Answer _____

_____

What part of the Kreb's cycle yields a high amount of energy, requires the presence of oxygen, and is the most efficient?

(A) Aerobic metabolism
(B) Anaerobic metabolism
(C) Glycolysis
(D) Ischemia

Your Answer _____

_____

Correct Answers

A–210

911

(A) Shock is a state of inadequate tissue perfusion.

A–211

(A) Aerobic metabolism requires oxygen and is the most efficient. Anaerobic metabolism yields much less energy and results in toxic by-products, such as lactic acid.

Questions

A patient in decompensated shock can no longer

(A) maintain a normal pulse rate
(B) maintain afterload
(C) maintain preload
(D) maintain skin warmth

Your Answer _____

911

A complication of a closed wound that involves an extremity injury and causes significant edema and swelling in the deep tissue is called

(A) a closed fracture
(B) compartment syndrome
(C) a keloid
(D) Cushing's triad

Your Answer _____

Correct Answers

A–212

(C) A patient in decompensated shock can no longer maintain preload. The pulse rate and skin warmth change in patients with compensated shock. This includes an increase in pulse rate and the skin feeling cool to the touch because of shunting of blood to the body's core.

A–213

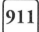

(B) Compartment syndrome is a complication of a closed wound, usually a crush injury. In this situation, an extremity injury causes progressive edema and swelling in the deep tissues. The pressure continues to rise in the injured extremity, causing neurovascular compromise. This is a serious condition requiring immediate medical attention.

Questions

911

Match each of the following terms to the correct definition.

Q–214 Abrasion

Q–215 Traumatic laceration

Q–216 Incision

Q–217 Puncture

Q–218 Avulsion

(A) Open wound with jagged edges
(B) Deep, narrow wound
(C) Scraping away of superficial layers of skin
(D) Tearing away of body tissue
(E) Smooth cut

Your Answer _____

_____

Correct Answers

$\boxed{911}$

A–214

(C)　An abrasion is the scraping or abrading away of superficial layers of the skin.

A–215

(A)　A traumatic laceration is an open wound with a tear or a jagged border.

A–216

(E)　An incision is a very smooth or surgical laceration typically caused by a knife, scalpel, razor blade, or piece of glass.

A–217

(B)　A puncture wound is a specific soft-tissue injury involving a deep, narrow wound to the skin and underlying organs that carries an increased risk of infection.

A–218

(D)　An avulsion is a forceful tearing away or separation of body tissue; an avulsion may be partial or complete.

Career Pulse

Paramedics get information by observing, receiving, and otherwise obtaining information from all relevant sources.

Questions

911

Which of the following is the proper sequence to control bleeding?

(A) Direct pressure, pressure point, elevation, tourniquet
(B) Tourniquet, elevation, pressure point, direct pressure
(C) Direct pressure, elevation, pressure point, tourniquet
(D) Elevation, direct pressure, pressure point, tourniquet

Your Answer _____

911

You cannot control bleeding and need to apply a tourniquet. You should do all the following EXCEPT

(A) write "TQ" on the patient's forehead
(B) release the tourniquet every 5 minutes
(C) tighten the tourniquet if bleeding continues
(D) monitor the patient

Your Answer _____

Correct Answers

A–219

911

(C) The appropriate sequence to control bleeding is to first apply direct pressure to the wound, typically using a dry dressing. If bleeding persists, you would elevate the body part to control the bleeding. If bleeding still persists, you would apply pressure at the pressure point for that part of the body. As a last resort, you would apply a tourniquet.

A–220

911

(B) Once you apply a tourniquet you should never loosen or remove it except under extraordinary circumstances.

Questions

911

You arrive on the scene of a patient whose left arm is amputated just below his elbow. Which of the following is the most appropriate care for the amputated arm?

(A) Place the amputated arm in a plastic bag, immerse the bag in cold water.

(B) Place the amputated arm in cool water.

(C) Place the amputated arm in a plastic bag and immerse the bag in ice.

(D) Cover the amputated arm in ice.

Your Answer _____

_____

911

Your patient has an ice pick stuck in the right eye. The most appropriate care for this patient would be to

(A) remove the ice pick and bandage the eye

(B) stabilize the ice pick with a paper cup and bandage that eye

(C) stabilize the ice pick with a paper cup and bandage both eyes

(D) do nothing except transport the patient immediately

Your Answer _____

_____

Correct Answers

A–221

911

(A) The most appropriate care for any amputated body part is to place it in a plastic bag and immerse the bag in cold water. You would then immediately transport the patient to the hospital.

A–222

911

(C) The best treatment for this patient is first to stabilize the ice pick in place using a bulky dressing. You can create a bulky dressing by placing a paper cup over the ice pick to cover the protruding part and then bandaging both eyes.

Questions

911

Which of the following objects can be removed?

(A) A knife impaled in a patient's chest
(B) An iron rod impaled in a patient's upper thigh
(C) A pencil impaled in a patient's hand
(D) A screwdriver impaled in a patient's cheek

Your Answer _____

Which of the following types of radiation can be stopped by paper?

(A) Alpha
(B) Beta
(C) Gamma
(D) Neutron

Your Answer _____

Correct Answers

A–223

911

(D) Given the information, the best possible answer is to remove the screwdriver from the patient's cheek. Objects in the cheek can be removed at times if it is interfering with airway control and the paramedic anticipates being able to control hemorrhaging with direct pressure. If the patient with the knife impaled in the chest, is in cardiac arrest and the knife is interfering with chest compressions, it is acceptable to remove the knife. Otherwise, impaled objects should not be removed but rather stabilized in place.

A–224

(A) Alpha radiation is the least potent of the four types of radiation. Paper or clothing can stop alpha rays. Beta rays can penetrate a few layers of clothing.

Questions

Which of the following is NOT a means to limit your exposure to radiation?

(A) Time
(B) Distance
(C) Shielding
(D) Type

Your Answer _____

In carbon monoxide poisoning, how many times greater is carbon monoxide's affinity for hemoglobin compared with oxygen's?

(A) 100
(B) 200
(C) 300
(D) 400

Your Answer _____

Correct Answers

A–225

(D) The amount of time you are exposed, the distance from the source, and shielding from the source are the three means to limit your exposure to radiation.

A–226

(B) Carbon monoxide's affinity for hemoglobin is 200 times greater than oxygen's affinity for hemoglobin.

Questions

911

Which of the following would you expect to see in a patient with partial-thickness burns?

(A) Red skin and pain at the site
(B) Skin hard to the touch
(C) Intense pain and blisters
(D) Little or no pain

Your Answer _____

911

Your patient has burns that involve the epidermis, dermis, fat, and muscle. These burns would be classified as

(A) full-thickness burns
(B) partial-thickness burns
(C) superficial burns
(D) none of the above

Your Answer _____

Correct Answers

A–227

$$\boxed{911}$$

(C) A patient with partial-thickness burns would have blisters, intense pain, and white-to-red skin that is moist and/or mottled. With superficial burns, a patient would have red skin and pain at the site. Full-thickness burns would result in charring, dark brown or white skin that is hard to the touch, and little or no pain except at the periphery of the burn.

A–228

$$\boxed{911}$$

(A) Full-thickness burns involve the epidermis, dermis, fat, and muscle. Partial-thickness burns involve the epidermis and dermis. Superficial burns involve only the epidermis.

Questions

$$\boxed{911}$$

Your patient is a 29-year-old female who has partial-thickness burns on both her hands and her abdomen. The total body surface area involved would be approximately

(A) 10%
(B) 13%
(C) 17%
(D) 27%

Your Answer _____

$$\boxed{911}$$

You are treating a 3-year-old male with burns to both legs, front and back. The total body surface involved is

(A) 36%
(B) 18%
(C) 27%
(D) 13.5%

Your Answer _____

Correct Answers

911

(B) The hands, front and back, are 2% each for a total of 4% for both hands, plus the abdomen, which is 9%. The total area would be 13%.

911

(C) Each leg on a child or infant is 13.5%. When both legs are involved, the total body surface is 27%.

Questions

911

Which of the following patients would NOT be a critical-burn patient?

(A) 22-year-old male with partial-thickness burns to the hands

(B) 33-year-old female with superficial burns to the anterior chest

(C) 16-year-old male with partial-thickness burns to the genitalia

(D) 21-year-old female with partial-thickness burns on the entire left leg

Your Answer _____

_____

911

You are treating a patient who was removed from a house fire. The patient does not appear to have any burns but does have a lot of soot on her face and body. You should be concerned about

(A) the patient's airway

(B) how to clean the soot from the patient

(C) the patient vomiting

(D) eschar

Your Answer _____

_____

Correct Answers

A–231

$\boxed{911}$

(B) Each of these patients would be critical except the 33-year-old female with superficial burns to the chest. Any burns to the face, hands, feet, joints, or genitalia or circumferential burns are critical burns.

A–232

$\boxed{911}$

(A) The major concern for a patient with soot on her face is the airway. This patient should receive high-flow oxygen and be closely monitored.

Questions

You arrive on the scene to find a patient with what appears to be electrical burns. An electrical wire is under the patient. The first thing you should do is

(A) remove the patient from the wire immediately
(B) use a wooden pole to remove the wire from the patient
(C) begin airway care to the patient
(D) make sure the wire is de-energized

Your Answer _____

911

You are treating a patient who was struck by lightning. The patient is unresponsive and not breathing. You check the pulse and find none. You apply the EKG monitor and find the patient to be in ventricular fibrillation. You should

(A) begin CPR
(B) control the airway by intubating
(C) defibrillate the patient
(D) recognize that you can do nothing for this patient

Your Answer _____

Correct Answers

A–233

(D) Scene safety is always your top priority. You should never touch a patient who has some connection to an electrical wire or try to remove the wire unless you are positive that the wire is de-energized. This may mean that you need to wait for the power company to arrive to ensure that the wire is de-energized.

A–234

(C) The most appropriate action would be to defibrillate the patient immediately and follow the advanced cardiac life support guidelines established by the American Heart Association.

Questions

Q–235

You arrive on the scene of a patient who is working at a fertilizer store. The patient was moving pallets of lime when one of the pallets got stuck and flipped over. Dry lime is everywhere, including on your patient. The patient is complaining of pain in the right leg and appears to have a tib-fib fracture. You should

(A) immobilize the leg
(B) wash the patient off with copious amounts of water
(C) brush off the dry lime gently
(D) brush off the dry lime and then rinse the rest of the lime off with water

Your Answer _____

Q–236

A partial displacement of a bone end from its position within a joint capsule is referred to as a

(A) sprain
(B) strain
(C) subluxation
(D) dislocation

Your Answer _____

Correct Answers

A–235

(D) The first step in caring for this patient would be decontamination. Water reacts with dry lime to create heat, causing burning of the skin. Therefore, you would want to gently brush off as much of the dry lime as possibly and then rinse the remainder of the lime from the patient's body with water. Once the patient is decontaminated, you would complete your assessment and begin the necessary treatment, such as immobilization of the injured leg.

A–236

(C) Subluxation is a partial displacement of a bone end from its position within a joint capsule. A sprain is a tearing of a joint capsule's connective tissues, typically a ligament. A strain occurs when muscle fibers are overstretched by forces that exceed the strength of the fibers. A dislocation is a complete displacement of bone ends from their normal position in the joint.

Questions

911

Match each of the following fractures to the correct definition.

Q–237   Transverse fracture

Q–238   Oblique fracture

Q–239   Comminuted fracture

Q–240   Spiral fracture

Q–241   Fatigue fracture

(A) A curving break in a bone that can be caused by rotational forces

(B) A break that runs across a bone, perpendicular to the bone's orientation

(C) A break in a bone associated with prolonged or repeated stress

(D) A break in a bone running across it at an angle other than 90 degrees

(E) A fracture in which the bone is broken into several pieces

Your Answer _____

_____

Correct Answers

A–237 to 241

911

A–237

(B) A transverse fracture is a break that runs across a bone, perpendicular to the bone's orientation.

A–238

(D) An oblique fracture is a break in a bone running across it at an angle other than 90 degrees.

A–239

(E) A comminuted fracture is a fracture in which the bone is broken into several pieces.

A–240

(A) A spiral fracture is a curving break in a bone that can be caused by rotational forces.

A–241

(C) A fatigue, or stress, fracture is a break in a bone associated with prolonged or repeated stress.

Career Pulse

Paramedics operate vehicles, mechanized devices, or equipment. They develop the skills needed for the running, maneuvering, navigating, or driving of vehicles or mechanized equipment, such as forklifts, passenger vehicles, aircraft, or watercraft.

Questions

Cushing's reflex is a sign of brain injury. The characteristics of this syndrome are

(A) increasing blood pressure, slowing pulse, and erratic respirations

(B) decreasing blood pressure, increasing pulse, and slow respirations

(C) increasing blood pressure, slowing pulse, and slow respirations

(D) decreasing blood pressure, slowing pulse, and fast respirations

Your Answer _____

Your patient is complaining of right-side weakness. You notice that her face is drooping on the left side. She is having difficulty speaking and appears to be drooling. She is hypertensive and seems to be confused. You would suspect that this patient is having

(A) insulin shock

(B) a stroke

(C) an epidural hematoma

(D) seizures

Your Answer _____

Correct Answers

A–242

(A) Cushing's reflex is characterized by increasing blood pressure, slowing pulse, and erratic respirations.

A–243

(B) The signs and symptoms this patient is experiencing are consistent with a stroke.

Questions

Your patient is having her second seizure in less than 1 minute and did not regain consciousness between the seizures. The most appropriate treatment for this patient is to administer

(A) flumazenil
(B) Valium
(C) dextrose 50%
(D) Dilantin

Your Answer _____

Your patient is a 54-year-old female. She is very irritable and is acting odd. Her pulse is weak and rapid. Your assessment reveals a glucose level of 42. You would suspect

(A) hyperglycemia
(B) diabetic ketoacidosis
(C) hypoglycemia
(D) cerebral vascular accident

Your Answer _____

Correct Answers

A–244

(B) The most appropriate treatment for this patient is to administer 5–10 mg of Valium IVP. Flumazenil is an antidote for a Valium overdose. You would only give dextrose if the patient is hypoglycemic based on a fingerstick glucose reading. Dilantin is typically not given in the field.

A–245

(C) This patient has the classic signs and symptoms of hypoglycemia.

Questions

Which of the following is the most appropriate treatment for hypoglycemia in an adult?

(A) Dextrose 50%
(B) Dextrose 25%
(C) Insulin
(D) 100 mg thiamine

Your Answer _____

Your patient is complaining of shortness of breath. You notice he has urticaria over his entire body. He cannot talk very well, appears cool and clammy, and has low blood pressure. The most appropriate treatment for this patient would be administering high-flow oxygen and then epinephrine at which dosage?

(A) 0.1 to 0.35 mg of 1:1,000 solution IM
(B) 0.1 to 0.35 mg of 1:10,000 solution IVP
(C) 1 mg of 1:10,000 solution IVP
(D) 1 mg of 1:1,000 solution IM

Your Answer _____

Correct Answers

A–246

(A) One ampule of dextrose 50% is the most appropriate treatment for this patient. Administering insulin is typically never done in the field and is not within the paramedic's scope of practice. Thiamine should be given in alcoholic or malnourished patients along with dextrose for hypoglycemia.

A–247

(B) After administering high-flow oxygen (be prepared to manage airway with an advanced airway), you would give this patient epinephrine 0.1 to 0.35 mg 1:10,000 solution IVP. This patient is probably having a severe allergic reaction or anaphylaxis.

Questions

You respond to a local store that sells fertilizers. When you arrive on the scene, you find a 38-year-old male sitting outside. He is sweating and has tears running down his face. He appears to be incontinent and has defecated very loose stools. He complains of blurred vision. On examining the patient, you notice he has constricted pupils and is tachycardic.

Q–248

You would suspect that this patient is suffering from

(A) shock
(B) carbon monoxide poisoning
(C) organophosphate poisoning
(D) cyanide poisoning

Your Answer _____

_____

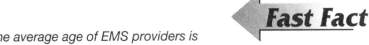

Fast Fact

The average age of EMS providers is about 35 for both EMTs and paramedics.

Correct Answers

A–248

(C) This patient displays the signs and symptoms of organophosphate poisoning. Many fertilizers are organophosphates.

Career Pulse

Paramedics are responsible for equipment maintenance. They perform routine maintenance on equipment and determine when and what kind of adjustments are needed.

Questions

Which of the following is the most appropriate sequence of treatment for this patient?

(A) Oxygen, decontamination, atropine 2–5 mg IVP
(B) Oxygen, atropine 1 mg IVP, decontamination
(C) Decontamination, oxygen, atropine 1 mg IVP
(D) Decontamination, oxygen, atropine 2–5 mg IVP

Your Answer _____

Which of the following is neurotoxic?

(A) Rattlesnake
(B) Coral snake
(C) Copperhead
(D) King snake

Your Answer _____

Correct Answers

(D) The first step in treating any patient who has been contaminated is decontamination. This is followed by administration of high-flow oxygen at 15 LPM through a nonrebreather mask. You may also need to consider intubation or assisting ventilation for this patient. Atropine is given at a higher dosage as an antidote for organophosphate-poisoning patients.

(B) The venom of the coral snake is a neurotoxin. The rattlesnake and copperhead are hemotoxic. The king snake is not poisonous.

Questions

Which of the following classifications of drugs causes psychosis, nausea, dilated pupils, rambling speech, head-ache, dizziness, and distortion of sensory perceptions?

(A) Barbiturates
(B) Narcotics
(C) Amphetamines
(D) Hallucinogens

Your Answer _____

Q–252 to 254

Match each of the following terms to the correct definition.

Q–252 Conduction

Q–253 Convection

Q–254 Radiation

(A) Transfer of heat through currents in liquids or gases
(B) Transfer of energy through space or matter
(C) Moving electrons, ions, heat, or sound waves through a medium

Your Answer _____

Correct Answers

A–251

(D) These are classic signs of hallucinogens. Another effect of these drugs is hallucinations.

A–252 to 254

A–252
(C) Conduction is the movement of electrons, ions, heat, or sound waves through a conductor or conducting medium.

A–253
(A) Convection is the transfer of heat via currents in liquids or gases.

A–254
(B) Radiation is the transfer of energy through space or matter.

Questions

You are treating a female patient who presents to you with confusion. Her respirations are deep and rapid, and her pulse is fast. She is also hypotensive. Her skin feels very hot to the touch, and she appears to be dry. You would suspect

(A) heat cramps
(B) heat exhaustion
(C) heat stroke
(D) hypothermia

Your Answer _____

Which of the following is NOT a major type of schizo-phrenia?

(A) Paranoid
(B) Catatonic
(C) Disorganized
(D) Differentiated

Your Answer _____

Correct Answers

(C) This patient is probably suffering from heat stroke. This is a true emergency, and this patient needs immediate cooling measures. Be prepared for seizures and possible cardiac arrest.

(D) The four major types of schizophrenia are paranoid, catatonic, disorganized, and undifferentiated. A patient with paranoid schizophrenia is preoccupied, has feelings of persecution, and may suffer delusions or auditory hallucinations. Disorganized schizophrenia causes the patient to display disorganized behavior, dress, or speech. Catatonic schizophrenia is evident when the patient exhibits catatonic rigidity, immobility, stupor, and/or peculiar voluntary movements. A patient with undifferentiated schizophrenia does not readily fit into one of the other categories.

Questions

Q–257

Which of the following is NOT a risk factor for suicide?

(A) Previous attempts
(B) Age
(C) Divorced or widowed
(D) Suicide of opposite-sexed parent

Your Answer _____

Q–258

You have just delivered a newborn. The baby appears pink with blue extremities, pulse rate is 102, respiratory effort is a strong cry, and the infant is moving actively. What is the infant's APGAR score?

(A) 10
(B) 9
(C) 8
(D) 7

Your Answer _____

Correct Answers

A–257

(D) The risk factors for suicide are previous attempts, depression, age, alcohol or drug abuse, being divorced or widowed, giving away personal items, living alone, homosexuality, major separation trauma, major physical stress, loss of independence, lack of goals and plans for the future, suicide of same-sexed parent, expression of a plan for committing suicide, and possession of the mechanism to commit suicide.

A–258

(B) Appearance scores a 1 because of the peripheral cyanosis, and pulse rate, grimace, activity, and respiratory rate each score a 2; therefore, the total score is 9.

Questions

The following scenario applies to questions 259 and 260.

You deliver a baby and notice a greenish stain on the newborn.

Q–259

This is known as
(A) amniotic fluid
(B) meconium stain
(C) uterine rupture
(D) dystocia

Your Answer _____

Q–260

What is the priority order for the steps in the most appropriate treatment for this infant?
I.   Dry the infant
II. Suction the nose
III. Oxygenate the infant
IV. Suction the mouth

(A) IV, II, III, I   (C) II, IV, III, I
(B) I, II, III, IV   (D) I, II, IV, III

Your Answer _____

Correct Answers

A–259

(B)   A yellowish green, light green, or dark green stain on a newborn is caused by meconium. This occurs when the infant makes its first bowel movement in the amniotic fluid. This can be a critical situation.

A–260

(A)   The steps in the most appropriate treatment for this infant are to first suction the mouth and then suction the nose. Because babies are nose breathers, if you suction the nose first, the baby will aspirate the meconium fluid and is thus highly likely to suffer morbidity or mortality.

Questions

You examine your patient who is full term in her pregnancy. She is delivering her baby breech. The head is still in the birth canal. You should

(A) place two fingers in the "V" position in the vaginal wall to allow the baby to breathe
(B) assist the mother in delivering the head
(C) immediately transport
(D) make a small incision in the perineum and continue the delivery

Your Answer _____

Which of the following is NOT a true statement?

(A) Albuterol is a sympathomimetic drug.
(B) Cardiac dysrhythmias associated with bradycardia are a contraindication to the administration of albuterol.
(C) Beta-blockers may antagonize albuterol.
(D) Albuterol relaxes the smooth muscles of the bronchial tree.

Your Answer _____

Correct Answers

A–261

(A) This is the only time it is permissible to insert anything in the vagina. In this situation, you need to place your fingers in a "V" position to allow the infant to breathe and then immediately transport the patient. Do not attempt to deliver this baby.

A–262

(B) Cardiac dysrhythmias associated with tachycardia are a contraindication to the administration of albuterol.

Questions

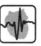

Which class of drug is atropine?

(A) Anticholinergic agent
(B) Beta-blocking agent
(C) Inotropic vasodilator
(D) Coronary vasodilator

Your Answer _____

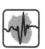

The maximum dose of diazepam is

(A) 5 mg
(B) 10 mg
(C) 20 mg
(D) 30 mg

Your Answer _____

Correct Answers

A–263

(A) Atropine is classified as an anticholinergic agent.

A–264

(D) Diazepam is given in 5- to 10-mg increments. The maximum dosage for adults is 30 mg.

Questions

Q–265

Which of the following is NOT an indication for Cardizem?

(A) Atrial fibrillation
(B) Atrial flutter
(C) Ventricular fibrillation
(D) Paroxysmal supraventricular tachycardia (PSVT)

Your Answer _____

Q–266

Which of the following doses of dopamine is a cardiac dose?

(A) 2–4 mcg/kg/min
(B) 5–10 mcg/kg/min
(C) 10–20 mcg/kg/min
(D) 20–25 mcg/kg/min

Your Answer _____

Correct Answers

A–265

(C) Cardizem is indicated in atrial fibrillation, atrial flutter, PSVT, and multifocal atrial tachycardias.

A–266

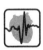

(B) A low dose, or renal dose, is 2–4 mcg/kg/min; a moderate dose, or a cardiac dose, is 5–10 mcg/kg/min; and 10–20 mcg/kg/min is a high dose, or vasopressor dose.

Questions

Which of the following is NOT an adverse reaction of diphenhydramine (Benadryl)?

(A) Hypersensitivity
(B) Palpitations
(C) Hypotension
(D) Dry mouth and throat

Your Answer _____

Which of the following is NOT a true statement about drug interactions for epinephrine?

(A) MAO inhibitors may potentiate the effect of epinephrine.
(B) Alpha-adrenergic antagonists may blunt the inotropic response to epinephrine.
(C) Sympathomimetics and phosphodiesterase inhibitors may exacerbate the dysrhythmia response to epinephrine.
(D) Epinephrine may be deactivated by alkaline solutions.

Your Answer _____

Correct Answers

A–267

(A) Hypersensitivity is a contraindication to administering diphenhydramine (Benadryl), not an adverse reaction.

A–268

(B) Beta-adrenergic antagonists may blunt the inotropic response to epinephrine, not alpha-antagonists.

Questions

Which of the following is the correct dose of epinephrine for a pediatric patient having a mild anaphylactic reaction?

(A) 0.3 mg of 1:1,000 solution IM
(B) 0.1 mL/kg of 1:1,000 solution IM
(C) 0.01 mL/kg of 1:1,000 solution IM
(D) 0.01 mg of 1:1,000 solution IM

Your Answer _____

_____

Furosemide is a potent diuretic that

(A) stimulates the reabsorption of sodium and chloride in the proximal tubule and loop of Henle
(B) inhibits the reabsorption of sodium and chloride in the proximal tubule and loop of Henle
(C) increases cardiac preload by increasing venous capacitance
(D) reduces cardiac preload by decreasing venous capacitance

Your Answer _____

_____

Correct Answers

A–269

(C) The correct dose for a pediatric patient having a mild anaphylactic reaction is 0.01 mL/kg of 1:1,000 dilution IM. For a moderate or severe reaction, the correct dose would be 0.05 mcg/kg/min of 1:1,000 solution IV.

A–270

(B) Furosemide is a potent diuretic that inhibits the re-absorption of sodium and chloride in the proximal tubule and loop of Henle. IV doses can also reduce cardiac pre-load by increasing venous capacitance.

Questions

Q–271

In which of the following arrhythmias is lidocaine NOT indicated?

(A) Ventricular tachycardia
(B) Ventricular fibrillation
(C) Wide complex tachycardia of uncertain origin
(D) Bigeminy at a rate of 80

Your Answer _____

Q–272

Which of the following is NOT an indication for magnesium sulfate?

(A) Seizures
(B) Status asthmaticus not responsive to beta-adrenergic drugs
(C) Suspected hypomagnesemia
(D) Torsades de pointes

Your Answer _____

Correct Answers

A–271

(D) Bigeminy at the rate of 80 is a bradycardic rhythm. Lidocaine could eliminate the premature ventricular contractions in a bigeminy rhythm, which in this case would result in a heart rate of 40 and a more unstable rhythm. You would need to increase the heart rate before administering lidocaine.

A–272

(A) Magnesium sulfate is indicated only in eclampsia patients with seizures, not every patient who has seizures.

Questions

Which of the following is NOT a contraindication to administering Alupent?

(A) Hypersensitivity
(B) Cardiac dysrhythmias
(C) Tachycardia caused by digitalis toxicity
(D) Bradycardia caused by digitalis toxicity

Your Answer _____

You are preparing to intubate a patient. To sedate the patient, you are ordered to use Versed. What is the maximum dosage for your 75-kg 38-year-old male patient?

(A) 0.5 mg
(B) 0.75 mg
(C) 2.5 mg
(D) 7.5 mg

Your Answer _____

Correct Answers

A–273

(D)   Bradycardia caused by digitalis toxicity is not a contraindication to administering Alupent.

A–274

(D)   The correct dose of Versed varies from 0.05 to 0.1 mg/kg. Therefore, the maximum dosage for this patient is 0.1 mg/kg × 75 kg = 7.5 mg.

Questions

Morphine is classified as a

(A) beta-blocking agent
(B) opioid analgesic
(C) anesthetic
(D) opioid antagonist

Your Answer _____

Nitroglycerin works by

(A) reducing the preload and decreasing the workload of the heart
(B) increasing the afterload and decreasing the workload of the heart
(C) increasing the workload of the heart and lowering the myocardial oxygen demand
(D) constricting the arterioles and veins

Your Answer _____

Correct Answers

A–275

(B) Morphine sulfate is an opioid analgesic. Narcan, which is the antidote for morphine, is an opioid antagonist.

A–276

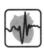

(A) Nitroglycerin dilates arterioles and veins in the periphery. It reduces the preload and, by reducing the afterload, decreases the workload of the heart and lowers myocardial oxygen demand.

Questions

Which of the following is a calcium channel blocker?

(A) Vasopressin
(B) Adenosine
(C) Verapamil
(D) Digoxin

Your Answer _____

_____

What is the correct dosage for vasopressin?

(A) 40 mg
(B) 40 units
(C) 40 mcg
(D) 40 g

Your Answer _____

_____

Correct Answers

(C) Verapamil is a calcium channel blocker.

(B) The correct dosage for vasopressin is 40 units IV push.

Questions

A P wave on an EKG strip represents

(A) atrial depolarization
(B) repolarization of the right and left ventricles
(C) depolarization of the right and left ventricles
(D) atrial repolarization

Your Answer _____

You see an elevation of the ST segment in leads II, III, and aVF. Which one of the following would you suspect?

(A) Septal wall infarct
(B) Anterior wall infarct
(C) Right ventricle infarct
(D) Inferior wall infarct

Your Answer _____

Correct Answers

A–279

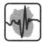

(A) P waves represent atrial depolarization. Repolarization of the right and left ventricles is represented by the ST segment. QRS complex represents depolarization of the right and left ventricles.

A–280

(D) An ST segment elevation in leads II, III, and aVF is highly suggestive of an inferior wall infarct.

Questions

A patient having a lateral wall infarct would typically have ST segment elevation in leads

(A) V1 and V2
(B) V3 and V4
(C) I, aVL, V5, and V6
(D) V4, V5, and V6

Your Answer _____

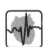

Your patient is complaining of chest pain. You attach the EKG monitor and see a tachycardic rhythm. You notice JVD, and his heart sounds are muffled. The patient's pulse pressure seems to be narrowing. You would suspect

(A) pulmonary edema
(B) cardiac tamponade
(C) pneumothorax
(D) cardiac contusion

Your Answer _____

Correct Answers

A–281

(C) A lateral wall infarct is indicated by an elevated ST segment in leads I, aVL, V5, and V6.

A–282

(B) This patient has the signs and symptoms of cardiac tamponade. This condition occurs when fluids leak into the pericardial sac, compressing the heart and preventing blood return. This can lead to cardiac arrest if untreated.

Questions

Your patient is complaining of tearing chest pain that radiates straight through to his back. His pulse is 96. He appears cool, clammy, and pale. The patient states that this condition came on suddenly. He denies any other symptoms at this point. This patient is most likely suffering from

(A) myocardial infarction
(B) pulled chest muscle
(C) pneumonia
(D) aortic dissection

Your Answer _____

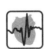

Your patient is complaining of shortness of breath. She has pink, frothy sputum. Her blood pressure is low. She is cool and clammy to the touch. You would suspect

(A) right-sided heart failure
(B) left-sided heart failure
(C) pneumonia
(D) myocardial infarction

Your Answer _____

Correct Answers

A–283

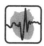

(D) This patient is most likely suffering from an aortic dissection. The classic sign is the tearing pain radiating directly to the back.

A–284

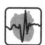

(B) This patient is probably having left-sided heart failure. The left side of the heart is not functioning properly, and the blood is beginning to back up. She develops fluid in her lungs that she coughs up as a pink, frothy sputum.

Questions

A patient having an anterior wall infarct would typically have ST segment elevation in leads

(A) V1 and V2
(B) V3 and V4
(C) I, aVL, V5, and V6
(D) V4, V5, and V6

Your Answer _____

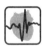

A patient having a septal wall infarct would typically have ST segment elevation in leads

(A) V1 and V2
(B) V3 and V4
(C) I, aVL, V5, and V6
(D) V4, V5, and V6

Your Answer _____

Correct Answers

A–285

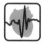

(B) A patient having an anterior wall infarct would typically have ST segment elevation in leads V3 and V4.

A–286

(A) A patient having a septal wall infarct would have ST segment elevation in leads V1 and V2.

Questions

Which of the following is an absolute contraindication to administering a fibrinolytic agent to a patient with myocardial infarction?

(A) Chest pain for 20 minutes
(B) History of an intracranial bleed
(C) Under 75 years of age
(D) Less than 12 hours since the onset of symptoms

Your Answer _____

_____

Q–288

911

Your patient appears to have a head injury. A witness said that the patient lost consciousness and then completely regained consciousness. Now, the patient is complaining of a severe headache and appears to be getting progressively confused. This patient is most likely suffering from a(n)

(A) subdural hematoma
(B) epidural hematoma
(C) subarachnoid hemorrhage
(D) cerebral hematoma

Your Answer _____

_____

Correct Answers

A–287

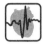

(B) The absolute contraindications to administering fibrinolytic agents are history of intracranial bleeding or hemorrhagic stroke, nonhemorrhagic stroke within 1 year, internal bleeding, and suspected aortic dissection.

A–288

(B) This patient is most likely suffering from an epidural hematoma. The loss of consciousness followed by regaining consciousness (lucid interval) and then progressive decline is typical of the condition.

Questions

Q–289

911

Your patient was involved in a diving injury. The patient is complaining of no feeling from the nipple line down. You would suspect a spinal injury at

(A) T4
(B) C7
(C) T10
(D) L1

Your Answer _____

_____

Q–290

911

Which of the following is NOT a sign or symptom of a pulmonary contusion?

(A) Tachypnea
(B) Bradycardia
(C) Apprehension
(D) Hemoptysis

Your Answer _____

_____

Correct Answers

A–289

911

(A)   No sensation or motor function from the nipple line down typically indicates an injury at T4.

A–290

911

(B)   The signs and symptoms of a pulmonary contusion are tachypnea, tachycardia, apprehension, hemoptysis, cough, respiratory distress, dyspnea, evidence of blunt trauma, and cyanosis.

Questions

911

The rate and depth of breathing will increase with

(A) acidosis
(B) alkalosis
(C) narcotic overdoses
(D) myasthenia gravis

Your Answer _____

_____

911

You are preparing for a long-distance transport. The patient is on 12 LPM of oxygen. You have 1,800 L of oxygen left in your on-board M cylinder oxygen tank. How long will this tank last at a rate of 12 LPM?

(A) 120 minutes
(B) 150 minutes
(C) 208 minutes
(D) 416 minutes

Your Answer _____

_____

Correct Answers

A–291

911

(A)   The rate and depth of breathing will increase with acidosis, anxiety, aspirin poisoning, oxygen need, pain, and lesions in the central nervous system (pons).

A–292

911

(C)   You first subtract 200 L (safe residual) from 1,800 L, which yields 1,600 L. You then use the factor for the M cylinder, which is 1.56: 1,600 L × 1.56, which yields 2,496 L. You then divide 2,496 L by 12 LPM, which gives you 208 min, or almost 3.5 hours.

Questions

911

You are delivering 6 LPM of oxygen via nasal cannula. You are delivering approximately what percentage of oxygen?

(A) 24%
(B) 44%
(C) 35%
(D) 60%

Your Answer _____

911

Adult patients should be suctioned no longer than

(A) 5 seconds
(B) 15 seconds
(C) 30 seconds
(D) 1 minute

Your Answer _____

Correct Answers

A–293

911

(B) A nasal cannula flowing at 6 LPM delivers approximately 44% oxygen.

A–294

911

(B) An adult patient should be suctioned no longer than 15 seconds.

Questions

Pediatric patients should be suctioned no longer than

(A) 5 seconds
(B) 15 seconds
(C) 30 seconds
(D) 1 minute

Your Answer _____

You need to select an endotracheal tube for your 4-year-old patient. Which of the following would be the best tube size for this patient?

(A) 4.0 ET cuffed
(B) 4.0 ET uncuffed
(C) 5.0 ET cuffed
(D) 5.0 ET uncuffed

Your Answer _____

Correct Answers

A–295

(A) Pediatric patients should be suctioned no longer than 5 seconds.

A–296

(D) A 5.0 ET uncuffed is the best tube size for this patient. You determine this by dividing the patient's age by 4 and then adding 4. Uncuffed tubes are preferred for children under the age of 8.

Questions

Q–297

911

Your patient has a chronic reduction in arterial Po^2 and an increased red blood cell production known as polycythemia. With which condition is the elevation of hematocrit or polycythemia most seen?

(A) Emphysema
(B) Chronic bronchitis
(C) Both A and B
(D) Neither A nor B

Your Answer _____

Q–298

Your patient is thin and has a barrel chest. He states he has not had a productive cough, but you hear wheezing and rhonchi. The patient has a pink complexion and appears to be having significant trouble breathing. When he inhales, he is pursing his lips. You would suspect that this patient has

(A) tuberculosis
(B) chronic bronchitis
(C) emphysema
(D) CHF

Your Answer _____

Correct Answers

911

(B) This is more common in patients with chronic bronchitis ("blue bloater" patients) than in those with emphysema ("pink puffer" patients).

(C) This patient has all the classic signs of emphysema.

Questions

Your patient is a 22-year-old female. She is complaining of a sudden onset of pain in her chest, predominately on her left side. She states it is very sharp and worse with inspiration. The only medication she takes is birth control pills, and she is a smoker. She has no other significant history. You would suspect

(A) myocardial infarction
(B) tension pneumothorax
(C) asthma
(D) pulmonary embolism

Your Answer _____

The incident command system is built around five major components. Which of the following is NOT a major component?

(A) Planning
(B) Medical
(C) Operations
(D) Logistics

Your Answer _____

Correct Answers

A–299

(D) This patient is most likely suffering from a pulmonary embolism. The risk of pulmonary embolism goes up with the use of birth control pills and smoking.

A–300

(B) Medical is part of operations but not a major component. The five components are command, planning, operations, logistics, and finance.

Questions

The following scenario applies to questions 301 and 302.

Your patient appears to be very anxious. She is taking about 60 breaths a minute. She tells you she is having chest pain with tingling down both her arms and up into her face.

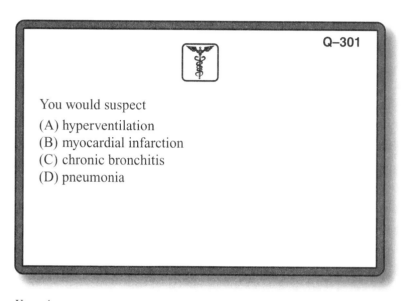

Q–301

You would suspect

(A) hyperventilation
(B) myocardial infarction
(C) chronic bronchitis
(D) pneumonia

Your Answer _____

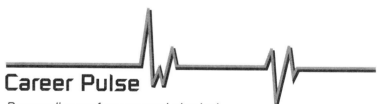

Career Pulse

Paramedics perform general physical activities such as climbing, lifting, balancing, walking, stooping, and handling of materials.

Correct Answers

A–301

(A)   This patient is most likely suffering from hyperventilation.

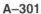

Career Pulse

Paramedics are responsible for keeping up-to-date technically and for applying any new knowledge to the job.

Questions

You would treat this patient by

(A) having her breathe into a paper bag

(B) providing high-flow oxygen through a nonrebreather mask

(C) coaching breathing

(D) assisting with a bag valve mask

Your Answer _____

Which of the following is an example of unified command?

(A) Affecting more than one political jurisdiction

(B) Involving multiple agencies within a jurisdiction

(C) Having an impact on multiple geographic and functional agencies

(D) All of the above

Your Answer _____

Correct Answers

A–302

(C) You should assist this patient by providing breath coaching. It works best if you mimic how you want the patient to breathe.

A–303

(D) All of these are examples of unified command, in which one agency is not reliant on outside agencies. Typically, unified command is used for short-duration incidents.

Questions

Which unit is responsible for communicating with hospitals to determine capabilities?

(A) Transportation
(B) Incident command
(C) Treatment
(D) Logistics

Your Answer _____

_____

Q–305

A low-head dam can

(A) create a dangerous hydraulic
(B) cause rip currents
(C) create a small overflow
(D) range from 12 inches to 20 feet

Your Answer _____

_____

Correct Answers

A–304

(A) One of the responsibilities of the transportation unit is to determine the capabilities of each receiving hospital.

A–305

(A) A low-head dam can range in height from 6 inches to 10 feet and can create a dangerous hydraulic.

Questions

There are seven phases of a rescue operation. The correct order of these phases is

(A) arrival and scene size-up, gaining access to the patient, disentanglement, medical treatment, hazard control, patient packaging, transportation

(B) arrival and scene size-up, hazard control, gaining access to the patient, medical treatment, disentanglement, patient packaging, transportation

(C) arrival and scene size-up, hazard control, disentanglement, gaining access to the patient, patient packaging, medical treatment, transportation

(D) arrival and scene size-up, disentanglement, gaining access to the patient, medical treatment, patient packaging, hazard control, transportation

Your Answer _____

_____

Fast Fact

There are currently more men in EMS than women. Men make up about 70% of paramedics and about 59% of EMTs. There are, however, more female EMTs than female paramedics.

Correct Answers

A–306

(B) The correct order of the seven phases of a rescue operation is (1) arrival and scene size-up, (2) hazard control, (3) gaining access to the patient, (4) medical treatment, (5) disentanglement, (6) patient packaging, and (7) transportation.

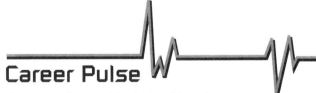

Career Pulse

A paramedic must be trained to enter, transcribe, record, store, or maintain information in written or electronic form.

Questions

You are at the scene of a hazardous materials incident. You are told that personnel need to be in the highest level of personal protective equipment (PPE). The highest level of PPE is

(A) level A
(B) level B
(C) level C
(D) level D

Your Answer _____

911

Which of the following types of chemical acts on the nervous system?

(A) Irritants
(B) Asphyxiants
(C) Anesthetics
(D) Nephrotoxins

Your Answer _____

Correct Answers

(A) The highest level of PPE is level A. Level D is the daily uniform.

(C) Anesthetics act on the nervous system by affecting either the cardiorespiratory-regulating mechanisms of the brain or the ability to transmit impulses required for adequate respiratory and circulatory functions.

Questions

911

Match each of the following terms to the correct definition.

Q–309 IDLH

Q–310 LD-50

Q–311 PEL

Q–312 Flash point

Q–313 Vapor density

Q–314 TLV-STEL

(A) The minimum temperature at which a liquid gives off enough vapors to ignite but not continue to burn

(B) The maximum time-weighted concentration at which 95% of exposed healthy adults suffer no adverse effects

(C) The dose that, when administered to laboratory animals, kills 50% of them

(D) A 15-minute time-weighted average exposure that should not be exceeded at any time and not repeated more than four times a day, with 60-minute rest periods required between each exposure

(E) Any atmosphere that poses an immediate hazard to life or produces immediate, irreversible, debilitating effects on health

(F) The weight of a pure vapor or gas compared with the weight of an equal volume of dry air at the same temperature

Your Answer _____

Correct Answers

911

A–309

(E) Immediately dangerous to life and health (IDLH) is any atmosphere that poses an immediate hazard to life or produces immediate, irreversible, debilitating effects on health.

A–310

(C) Lethal dose, 50% kill (LD-50) is the dose that, when administered to laboratory animals, kills 50% of them.

A–311

(B) Permissible exposure limit (PEL) is the maximum time-weighted concentration at which 95% of exposed healthy adults suffer no adverse effects.

A–312

(A) Flash point is the minimum temperature at which a liquid gives off enough vapors to ignite but not continue to burn.

A–313

(F) Vapor density is the ratio of the weight of a pure vapor or gas to the weight of an equal volume of dry air at the same temperature.

A–314

(D) Threshold limit value, short-term exposure limit (TLV-STEL) is a 15-minute time-weighted average exposure that should not be exceeded at any time and not repeated more than four times a day, with 60-minute rest periods required between each exposure.

Questions

The Ryan White Comprehensive AIDS Resources Emergency Act of 2009 requires that

(A) emergency responders report exposures to infectious diseases
(B) emergency responders be advised if they have been exposed to infectious diseases
(C) emergency responders be advised if they have been exposed to AIDS
(D) emergency responders report patients with AIDS

Your Answer _____

_____

Which of the following is NOT a defense to a negligence claim?

(A) Good Samaritan laws
(B) Personal immunity
(C) Statute of limitations
(D) Contributory negligence

Your Answer _____

_____

Correct Answers

A–315

(B) The Ryan White Comprehensive AIDS Resources Emergency Act of 2009 requires that emergency responders be advised if they have been exposed to infectious diseases, including hepatitis, tuberculosis, bacterial meningitis, rubella, and HIV.

A–316

(B) Good Samaritan laws, statutes of limitations, contributory negligence, and governmental immunity are defenses to negligence claims.

Questions

Q–317

Seven phases of communications occur during a typical EMS event. Which of the following is NOT one of the phases?

(A) Occurrence of the event
(B) Notification and emergency response
(C) Notification to the medical director
(D) Preparation of EMS for the next emergency response

Your Answer _____

Q–318

Which of the following is NOT a component of the narrative portion of the patient care report?

(A) Initial contact
(B) Pertinent oral statements
(C) Changes in patient status
(D) List of all crew members

Your Answer _____

Correct Answers

A–317

(C) The phases of communications that occur during a typical EMS event are (1) occurrence of the event, (2) detection of the need for emergency services, (3) notification and emergency response, (4) EMS arrival, (5) treatment, (6) preparation for transport, and (7) preparation of EMS for the next emergency response.

A–318

(D) The narrative portion of the patient care report contains initial contact, all patient care activities, initial assessment and vital signs, chief complaint, pertinent significant medical history, clock time of hospital contact, time of physician orders and advice, pertinent negative findings, pertinent oral statements, changes in patient status, patient response to treatment, vital sign reassessment, ECG interpretation, use of support services, time and condition of patient on delivery, and name of receiving health care worker. A list of all crew members goes elsewhere in the report.

Questions

Which of the following statements is NOT correct regarding correcting errors on a patient care report?

(A) Note the purpose of the revision or correction and why the information did not appear on the original document.

(B) Note the date and time the revision or correction was made.

(C) Ensure that the revision or correction was made by the original author of the document.

(D) Make the revision or correction as soon as the need for it is realized by blacking out any errors to avoid confusion.

Your Answer _____

_____

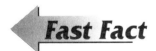

Requirements for certification as a paramedic differ from state to state.

Correct Answers

A–319

(D) You should make any revision or correction to a patient care report as soon as you realize it is necessary; however, you should draw a line through any words you wish to delete. Never black out any errors on the patient care report.

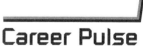

Career Pulse

A paramedic is responsible for providing information to supervisors, peers, or subordinates —by telephone, in printed form, e-mail, or in person.

Questions

Q–320

The initial assessment of a pediatric patient may be performed by using the pediatric assessment triangle. Which of the following assessments is NOT part of the pediatric assessment triangle?

(A) Respiratory depth size of chest wall
(B) Mental status for circulation
(C) Muscle tone for work of breathing
(D) Respiratory rate for appearance

Your Answer _____

_____

Q–321

You are called to a 3-year-old male who is having trouble breathing. He has a barking cough and is not drooling. The parents said his condition came on about 3 to 4 hours ago and does not seem to be getting better. He is running a fever of around 102°F. You would suspect

(A) croup
(B) epiglottitis
(C) asthma
(D) upper airway infection

Your Answer _____

_____

Correct Answers

A–320

(A) The pediatric assessment triangle comprises appearance—mental status and muscle tone, work of breathing—respiratory rate and effort, and circulation—skin signs and color.

A–321

(A) This patient has the classic signs of croup. Croup is most often found in patients aged 6 months to 4 years. The onset is slow, and the patient typically has a barking cough. The patient usually does not drool and runs a fever of under 104°F.

Questions

The following scenario applies to questions 322–324.

This condition refers to any disease of the heart muscle that causes a reduction in the force of heart contractions and a resultant decrease in the efficiency of circulation of blood throughout the lungs and to the rest of the body.

Q–322

What is the condition?

(A) Cardiogenesis

(B) Cardiogenic shock

(C) Cardiomyopathy

(D) Cardiorespiratory compromise

Your Answer _____

Fast Fact

Paramedics on average have approximately four to five more years of experience than EMTs.

Correct Answers

(C) This condition is cardiomyopathy.

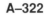

Career Pulse

The EMS and ambulance service's role during a natural disaster or public health emergency includes patient triage, decontamination, treatment, transport and disaster shelter staffing.

Questions

All the following signs and symptoms can be found in a pediatric patient with this condition EXCEPT

(A) fatigue
(B) chest pain
(C) conjunctivitis
(D) bradycardia

Your Answer _____

The treatment for this patient includes

(A) IV fluid therapy
(B) oxygen
(C) diuretics
(D) all of the above

Your Answer _____

Correct Answers

A–323

(C) Fatigue, chest pain, and dysrhythmias can be symptoms of cardiomyopathy.

A–324

(D) All the listed treatments are correct; however, the IV fluid therapy should be limited to avoid fluid overload.

Questions

You are treating a 5-year-old female who has inspiratory stridor and a fever of 105°F. She does not want to lie down. Her parents say that her symptoms came on suddenly. You would do all the following EXCEPT

(A) make no attempt to lay the patient down
(B) attempt to visualize her airway
(C) administer 100% oxygen
(D) do not start an IV

Your Answer _____

Your pediatric patient has a heart rate of less than 60. You are going to administer atropine. The correct dose for this patient is

(A) 0.01 mg/kg
(B) 0.02 mg/kg
(C) 0.03 mg/kg
(D) 0.05 mg/kg

Your Answer _____

Correct Answers

A–325

(B) This patient may be suffering from epiglottitis. The patient should be kept calm. You would not attempt to visualize the airway of the patient unless she needs ventilation assistance.

A–326

(B) The correct dosage for a pediatric patient is 0.02 mg/kg. The minimum dosage is 0.1 mg, and 0.5 mg is the maximum dose.

Questions

You are going to defibrillate a 4-year-old patient. The correct number of joules for the initial shock is

(A) 1 J/kg
(B) 2 J/kg
(C) 3 J/kg
(D) 4 J/kg

Your Answer _____

You are dispatched to a patient having seizures. You arrive on the scene to find an 18-month-old female actively seizing. When you touch the patient, she feels very hot. The parents say she has not been feeling well. You would suspect

(A) febrile seizures
(B) septic shock
(C) grand mal seizures
(D) head injury

Your Answer _____

Correct Answers

A–327

(B) The initial shock for a pediatric patient is 2 J/kg.

A–328

(A) The patient is most likely having febrile seizures. However, other types of seizures are possible and should be considered in your differential.

Questions

Q–329

You are directed to give your pediatric patient Valium rectally. The correct dosage via this route is

(A) 0.1 mg/kg
(B) 0.25 mg/kg
(C) 0.5 mg/kg
(D) 1 mg/kg

Your Answer _____

Q–330

Which of the following is NOT an indication for endotracheal intubation in neonatal resuscitation?

(A) Tracheal suctioning of meconium
(B) Tracheal administration of medications
(C) Effective bag-valve-mask ventilation
(D) Special resuscitation circumstances

Your Answer _____

Correct Answers

A–329

(C) A 0.5-mg/kg dose of Valium (higher than the oral dose) is required because absorption is incomplete when the drug is administered rectally.

A–330

(C) Endotracheal intubation is indicated in neonatal re-suscitation for tracheal suctioning of meconium, tracheal administration of medications, ineffective or prolonged bag-valve-mask ventilation, performance of chest compressions, and special resuscitation circumstances.

Questions

An inverted pyramid can be used to reflect the frequency of each skill used on neonates. Place the skills in the proper order from the top of the inverted pyramid to the bottom.

I.   Oxygen
II. Medications
III. Intubation
IV. Bag-valve-mask ventilation
V.   Position, suction, tactile stimulation
VI. Chest compressions

(A) I, II, III, IV, V, VI
(B) V, I, IV, VI, III, II
(C) I, IV, III, VI, V, II
(D) V, I, III, IV, II, VI

Your Answer _____

Fast Fact

Many communities are served by high-performance emergency ambulance service providers with proven track records in simultaneously delivering clinical excellence, response-time reliability, economic efficiency and customer satisfaction.

Correct Answers

A–331

(B) The inverted pyramid begins at the top with position, suction, tactile stimulation; oxygen; bag-valve-mask ventilation; chest compressions; intubation; and medications.

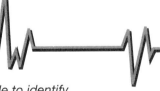

Career Pulse

Paramedics must be able to identify objects, actions, and events. They identify information by categorizing, estimating, recognizing differences or similarities, and detecting changes in circumstances or events.

Questions

Q–332

Which of the following statements is true?

(A) There are two umbilical arteries and one umbilical vein.

(B) There is one umbilical artery and two umbilical veins.

(C) There are two umbilical arteries and two umbilical veins.

(D) There is one umbilical artery and one umbilical vein.

Your Answer _____

Q–333

Chest compressions in neonates should be started when

(A) the heart rate is absent

(B) the heart rate is below 100

(C) the heart rate is below 60

(D) both A and C

Your Answer _____

Correct Answers

A–332

(A)   There are two umbilical arteries and one umbilical vein.

A–333

(D)   Chest compressions should be started on neonates when the heart rate drops below 60. If there is no heartbeat, compressions should also be started.

Questions

Which of the following should routinely be prevented in neonates?

(A) Vomiting
(B) Heat loss
(C) Hyperthermia
(D) Both B and C

Your Answer _____

You just delivered a baby. The mother admitted that she is addicted to morphine and may have taken some before the delivery. The neonate seems to be very lethargic with depressed respirations. To the newborn, you should administer

(A) 0.1 mg/kg of Narcan IVP
(B) 1.0 mg Narcan IVP
(C) 1.0 mg/kg Narcan IVP
(D) 0.1 mg Narcan IVP

Your Answer _____

Correct Answers

A–334

(B) Neonates tend to lose heat quickly. You should prevent heat loss and hypothermia. You typically do not need to worry about hyperthermia in neonates. You cannot prevent the neonate from vomiting, but you should protect the airway.

A–335

(A) You would administer 0.1 mg/kg of Narcan IVP to the newborn. The baby may have morphine in its system, and that may be the cause of the respiratory depression.

Questions

Which of the following is the correct dosage of dextrose for infants?

(A) 25 g of D50
(B) 25 g of D25
(C) 0.5 to 1.0 g/kg of D25
(D) 5 to 10 mL/kg of D25

Your Answer _____

Which of the following is NOT a major fear of school-age children?

(A) Loss of control
(B) The unknown and the dark
(C) Death
(D) Failure to live up to expectations of others

Your Answer _____

Correct Answers

(C) You can either administer 0.5 to 1.0 g/kg of D25 or 5 to 10 mL/kg of D10.

(B) Preschoolers have the fear of the unknown and the dark. School-age children tend to have fear of loss of control, death, failure to live up to expectations of others, bodily injury, and mutilation.

Questions

Which of the following statements is true?

(A) Bronchiolitis and asthma are the same illnesses, and both are characterized by wheezing.

(B) Bronchiolitis and asthma are different illnesses, but asthma is characterized by wheezing.

(C) Bronchiolitis and asthma are different illnesses, but both are characterized by wheezing.

(D) Bronchiolitis and asthma are the same illnesses, but asthma is characterized by wheezing.

Your Answer _____

With dehydration, which of the following is a severe amount of body weight loss in an infant?

(A) 5%

(B) 7%

(C) 10%

(D) 15%

Your Answer _____

Correct Answers

A–338

(C)   Bronchiolitis and asthma are different illnesses, but both are characterized by wheezing.

A–339

(D)   In an infant, 15% weight loss is severe, 10% is moderate, and 5% is mild.

Questions

Q–340

Your patient is a 3-year-old male who is hemorrhaging. The patient is tachypneic and combative. His extremities are cool, his blood pressure is normal, and he is tachycardic. You would classify this patient's hemorrhage as

(A) very mild
(B) mild
(C) moderate
(D) severe

Your Answer _____

Q–341

You are examining a 5-year-old patient. She has warm skin, she is bradycardic, and her blood pressure is 70/40. She has impaired neurological functions. You would suspect

(A) septic shock
(B) hemorrhagic shock
(C) anaphylactic shock
(D) neurogenic shock

Your Answer _____

Correct Answers

A–340

(B) This patient's hemorrhage would be classified as mild according to his signs and symptoms.

A–341

(D) This patient is most likely suffering from neurogenic shock. A patient with neurogenic shock may have a normal or bradycardic pulse and low blood pressure.

Questions

There are four goals of postresuscitation stabilization. Which of the following is NOT one of those goals?

(A) Preserve brain function

(B) Avoid primary organ injury

(C) Seek and correct causes of illness

(D) Enable the patient to arrive at an appropriate care facility in the best possible physiological state

Your Answer _____

_____

Which of the following is the most common cause of injury in children?

(A) Falls

(B) Motor vehicle accidents

(C) Pedestrian accidents

(D) Drowning

Your Answer _____

_____

Correct Answers

A–342

(B) Avoiding primary organ injury is not one of the four goals of postresuscitation stabilization. The correct fourth goal is avoiding secondary organ injury.

A–343

(A) Falls are the leading cause of injuries in children. Motor vehicles are the leading cause of death and serious injuries in children.

Questions

Q–344

Which of the following is the most common cause of death in pediatric patients?

(A) Chest injuries
(B) Spinal injuries
(C) Head injuries
(D) Abdominal injuries

Your Answer _____

Q–345

Which of the following statements about chest injuries in pediatric patients is true?

(A) Chest injuries in children under 14 years of age are usually the result of penetrating trauma.
(B) Tension pneumothorax is well tolerated in pediatric patients.
(C) Flail segments are relatively common in pediatric patients.
(D) Pediatric patients with cardiac tamponade may have no physical signs of tamponade other than hypotension.

Your Answer _____

Correct Answers

A–344

(C) Head injuries are the most common cause of death in pediatric trauma patients.

A–345

(D) Chest injuries in children under 14 years of age are usually the result of blunt trauma. Tension pneumothorax is poorly tolerated in pediatric patients. Flail segments are not common in pediatric patients.

Questions

Which of the following organs is (are) most commonly injured in pediatric patients?

(A) Liver
(B) Kidneys
(C) Spleen
(D) All of the above

Your Answer _____

You are treating a patient who is 10 years old. She has eyes that slope upward at the outer corners. Her tongue seems to be large and protruding. Her face is small and she has small facial features. You would suspect that this patient has

(A) Down syndrome
(B) anaphylactic reaction
(C) the signs of premature birth
(D) none of the above

Your Answer _____

Correct Answers

A–346

(D) The most common abdominal injuries in pediatric patients are those to the liver, kidneys, and spleen.

A–347

(A) This patient shows the classic signs of Down syndrome.

Questions

You are having difficulty starting an IV on a pediatric patient. You decide to place an intraosseous (IO) line. Which of the following is the proper placement of an IO line?

(A) In the epiphyseal plate
(B) Two finger breadths below the tibial tuberosity
(C) In the tibial tuberosity
(D) None of the above

Your Answer _____

Which of the following is NOT a contraindication to IO line placement?

(A) Fracture of the site or proximal to the site
(B) Cellulitis
(C) Burns that may be infected by the technique
(D) Poor venous access

Your Answer _____

Correct Answers

A–348

(B) The best location for an IO line is two finger breadths below the tibial tuberosity on the anteromedial surface of the tibia, directed away from the tibial growth plate.

A–349

(D) Poor venous access is one reason to start an IO line. In addition to those listed, other contraindications to starting an IO line include congenital bone disease and traumatized extremity.

Questions

Q–350

Which of the following is NOT a potential systemic complication in starting an IO line?

(A) Osteomyelitis
(B) Slow infusion from clotting of marrow
(C) Fat embolism
(D) Fracture

Your Answer _____

_____

Fast Fact

As their key role was demonstrated during the terror attacks of Sept. 11, 2001, ambulance providers are operating at a heightened state of readiness and are working to build the necessary capacity to respond to new homeland security threats such as bio-terrorism attacks.

Correct Answers

A–350

(B) Systemic complications include all the listed choices plus slight periostitis at the injection site and infection. Technical complications include slow infusion from clotting of marrow, subperiosteal infusion, and penetration of posterior wall of medullary cavity resulting in soft tissue infusion.

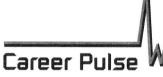

Career Pulse

The emergency medical services (EMS) system assures a timely and medically appropriate response to each request for out-of-hospital care and medical transportation, including emergency responses resulting from 9-1-1 calls and inter-facility transports.

Blank Cards for
Your Own Questions

Correct Answers

Blank Cards for
Your Own Questions

Correct Answers

INDEX

Note: Numbers in the Index refer to question numbers.

Braxton-Hicks contractions, 197
breech births, 259
ectopic pregnancy, 185
labor stages, 198–200
meconium stain, 260–261
placenta previa, 189–191
preeclampsia, 194–196
spontaneous abortions, 188
trauma patients, 187
Premature ventricular contractions
(PVCs), 180–181
Present illness, 63, 64
PSAP (Public Safety Answering
Point), 128
PSVT (paroxysmal supraventricular
tachycardia), 265
Public Safety Answering Point
(PSAP), 128
Pulmonary contusion, 290
Pulmonary edema, 33, 121
Pulmonary embolism, 145, 299
Pulse, 71, 114, 125
Pulseless electrical activity (PEA),
175–177
Punctures, 216
Pupils, 126
Purkinje system, 151
PVCs (premature ventricular
contractions), 180–181
Pyrogenic reactions, 35

R

Radial pulse, 75
Radiation
definition of, 254
limiting exposure, 225
types of, 224
Rales, 87
Rapid-sequence intubation, 56, 57
Red blood cells, 10, 26, 30
Renal failure, 85
Reports, patient care, 318, 319
Rescue operation, phases of, 305
Respiratory acidosis, 31
Respiratory alkalosis, 31
Respiratory rate, 82

Rhonchi, 45, 46, 89
Ryan White Comprehensive AIDS
Resources Emergency Act
(1990), 315

S

SA node, 149, 160
SaO_2 range, 47
Scene safety
domestic disputes, 105
and electrical wires, 233
motor vehicle accidents, 108
priorities for, 107
Scene size-up, 104
Schizophrenia, 256
Scope of practice, 2
Second-degree AV block type 1, 171
Seizures
febrile seizures, 328
in pregnant women with
preeclampsia, 196
treatment, 244, 272
Sellick maneuver, 48
Septal wall infarct, 286
Shock, 210, 212
Simplex communication systems,
129
Sinus bradycardia, 160–162
Sinus tachycardia, 163
Smooth muscle, 14
Snake bites, 250
Snoring, 45
Spinal injuries, 59, 289
Spiral fractures, 240
Spontaneous abortions, 188
Spontaneous pneumothorax, 146
Sprains, 236
Stoma, 61
Strains, 236
Striated (skeletal) muscle, 14
Stridor, 45, 46, 90
Strokes, signs/symptoms of, 243
Stroke volume, 203
Subluxation, 236
Suctioning, 62, 294–295
Suicide risk factors, 257

REFERENCES

American Heart Association Guidelines for Cardiopulmonary Resuscitation and Emergency Cardiovascular Care (multiple parts), *Circulation* 112, suppl. IV (2005).

Bledsoe, Bryan E., Robert S. Porter, and Richard A. Cherry, *Paramedic Care: Principles and Practice*, 2nd ed. (Upper Saddle River, NJ: Prentice Hall, 2005).

Sanders, Mick J. *Mosby's Paramedic Textbook*, 3rd ed. (St. Louis, MO: Mosby/JEMS, 2006).